MULTIDISCIPLINARY PUBLIC HEALTH

Understanding the development of the modern workforce

Jenny Wright, Fiona Sim and Katie Ferguson

First published in Great Britain in 2014 by

Policy Press
University of Bristol
6th Floor
Howard House
Queen's Avenue
Clifton
Bristol BS8 1SD
UK
Tel +44 (0)117 331 5020
Fax +44 (0)117 331 5367
e-mail pp-info@bristol.ac.uk
www.policypress.co.uk

North American office:
Policy Press
c/o The University of Chicago Press
1427 East 60th Street
Chicago, IL 60637, USA
t: +1 773 702 7700
f: +1 773-702-9756
e:sales@press.uchicago.edu
www.press.uchicago.edu

British Library Cataloguing in Publication Data
A catalogue record for this book is available from the British Library

Library of Congress Cataloging-in-Publication Data
A catalog record for this book has been requested

ISBN 978 1 44730 033 5 hardcover

Cover design by Qube Design Associates, Bristol
Front cover: www.istock.com
Printed and bound in Great Britain by CPI Group (UK) Ltd, Croydon, CR0 4YY
Policy Press uses environmentally responsible print partners

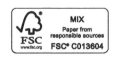

Contents

List of tables and figures

Tables

Figures

Acknowledgements

The authors are grateful to all those who have given so generously of their time in preparing this book, and in reflecting on the past and the whys and wherefores of what has been achieved. The authors had the privilege of talking to many people from the world of public health who had made substantial contributions to the achievements of the last 20 years. Some not only gave their time, but also shared their personal archives of documents relating to the multidisciplinary public health movement. The authors would particularly like to thank the following for their interest, time, insights and support in the writing of this book: John Ashton, Janet Baker, Jennie Carpenter, Jean Chapple, June Crown, Liam Donaldson, Selena Gray, Sue Gregory, Jenny Griffiths, Sian Griffiths, David Hunter, Tessa Lindfield, Jim McEwen, Klim McPherson, Maggie Pacini, Mala Rao, Cerilan Rogers, Paul Scourfield and Lillian Somervaille.

Our especial thanks go to Virginia Berridge for reading and commenting on the draft manuscript from the point of historical accuracy and presentation, also to Alison Firth, Royal Society for Public Health, for her help with the design of the map of the public health system, Figure 8.1.

The two witness seminars held in 2004 and 2005 – the first on the state of public health in the 1980s and 1990s and the second on the rise of the multidisciplinary public health movement from the 1990s to the early 2000s – were invaluable in providing insights to events as they unfolded. The third witness seminar, held in 2013, updated the account of the Health Protection Agency. The authors are also grateful to the Faculty of Public Health for access to their archive documents for relevant board and committee meetings and other papers.

The views expressed in the book are the authors' own.

About the authors

Jenny Wright has contributed to UK multidisciplinary public health since 2000 as a registered specialist, developing national competency and assessment frameworks and promoting public health careers. Between 1999 and 2004, Jenny was Chair of the Faculty of Public Health Medicine (FPHM) Honorary Members Committee, which then became the Specialist Development Committee.

Fiona Sim is currently Chair of the Royal Society for Public Health, Honorary Senior Lecturer at the London School of Hygiene and Tropical Medicine, Visiting Professor at the University of Bedfordshire, and a GP; she has contributed nationally to building public health capacity within service, research and the Department of Health (DH). A founding member of the Tripartite Group, representing the Royal Institute for Public Health (RIPH), she stood down from the group on taking up a role at DH in 2002.

Katie Ferguson is currently a Senior Public Health Officer in local government and is shortly to become a Public Health Speciality Registrar. Katie has a history doctorate and researched the multidisciplinary public health training scheme for her Masters in Public Health.

Foreword

by Sir Liam Donaldson

I started my public health training at a time when only doctors could do so. I had been working as a surgeon for several years, and it was quite a change. Very early in my transition, I became aware, of course, that medicine, and the medical model that I had been taught, explained only part of the public's health. Doctors and other health professionals have an important part to play in influencing the broader determinants of health and the system in which they work. But so, too, do many others.

When I became Chief Medical Officer for England, I strongly supported the notion that public health should not be the preserve of doctors – or, indeed, of any other single profession. Health is a complex interplay of many factors. The public's health is best improved by drawing on many different areas of expertise; therefore, public health needs to be multidisciplinary.

The public health workforce in England has shifted enormously in this direction over the last 15 years. The authors have done important work in studying and documenting this. Their findings make it clear that achieving this shift has not been easy. I hope that this book can serve as a reminder of this – so that what has been achieved can be built on further, and does not get lost.

ONE

Introduction and methods

Introduction

In the late 1990s, England embarked upon a journey to create a multidisciplinary public health workforce marked by equality of opportunity and equality of status at specialist level. This was in response to pressure, building from the late 1980s, from public health professionals from backgrounds other than medicine for recognition of their contribution to public health and for access to training and development. It was also in response to a better understanding of the changing public health needs of the time, which called for a broader range of skills in the workforce. The implications have been far-reaching and have led England to have a model for its public health workforce that is different from other developed countries. Although the stimulus was for recognition at specialist level, the ramifications of the changes that took place have embraced those involved in the operational delivery of public health services and have also led to consideration of the public health contribution made by the wider health and social care workforces.

Changing perceptions of public health

Public health, as a specific discipline, came to the fore in England during the 19th century in response to crises in sanitation and infection control leading to epidemics of typhoid and cholera, as well as high mortality rates. Medical Officers of Health, located within each local authority and heading up large teams of public health inspectors and nurses, led the implementation of a raft of legislation to improve sanitation, housing, food inspection and control of infectious diseases.[1]

Public health issues in the 21st century are very different from those perceived in the 19th century. Although a key area of work for

---

[1] The first Medical Officer of Health was appointed in 1847 in Liverpool. Two Public Health Acts (1848 and 1875) followed Edwin Chadwick's privately published report in 1842 on the poor sanitary conditions of the 'labouring population' of Great Britain. The Sanitary Acts of 1866–70 charged local authorities with responsibility for street clearing and for provision of sewers and clean water.

the public health workforce continues to be combating new and re-emerging infections (eg SARS[2] and influenza, respectively), much more attention is now devoted to reducing obesity, maintaining health in an ageing population, improving sexual health and tackling widening health inequalities in the face of recession.

There is no internationally agreed definition of public health. The Alma Ata Declaration (WHO and UNICEF, 1978), 'Health for all' (WHO, 1981) and the Ottawa Charter (WHO Europe, 1986) contain the modern emphasis on securing well-being as well as absence of disease. Public health was defined for the UK in 1988 by the then Chief Medical Officer (CMO) in his *Report of an inquiry into the future development of the public health function in England* (Acheson, 1988) as 'the science and art of preventing disease, prolonging life and promoting health through the organised efforts of society'. This built on an earlier definition by Winslow (1923), and was subsequently added to by Wanless (2004, p 23) in his second report on public health: 'through the organised efforts and informed choices of society, organisations, public and private, communities and individuals'. With this definition, therefore, public health has moved from being a relatively narrow discipline, based around a small professional workforce, to being the rightful consideration of the whole population – public health is, therefore, truly everyone's business. This book includes a section that reflects this so-called 'wider' public health workforce.

How the public health workforce has changed

As perceptions of what public health is and does have changed, so has the workforce needed to tackle the problems, as well as the skills needed within that workforce. Porter (1994), for example, in her introduction to 'The history of public health and the modern state', talks of public health as an eclectic mix of expert knowledge from the medical and social sciences. According to Lewis (1986, p 3), since the Second World War, public health, as a discipline, has 'allowed itself to become defined by the activities it undertook'. This was increasingly the case following the transfer of public health medical and nursing staff (along with the community health services for which they were responsible) from local authority employment to the National Health Service (NHS) in 1974, in a move to unite what was perceived as a dysfunctional split of health care responsibilities across the hospital, primary care and local authority sectors. Environmental health departments remained within

---

[2]   Severe Acute Respiratory Syndrome, identified in 2003.

local government, as well as other functions with a public health focus, such as housing, leisure, education and refuse collection.[3] Being located within the management and administrative tiers of the health service has meant that although they are able to influence service provision and commissioning through having prominent planning and strategic roles, much of the professional public health workforce has been subject to frequent reorganisation in line with frequent health service changes.

In line with the Coalition government's policy outlined in 2010 (DH, 2010b), the latest reorganisation (April 2013) has moved the vast majority of the health service public health workforce in England into either the civil service on the one hand, as part of a new national public health agency to strengthen the health protection response and population surveillance functions, or back into local government on the other, to focus primarily on improving health through a more effective, joined-up and locally accountable commissioning of programmes related to obesity, sexual health, physical activity, stopping smoking and improved physical and mental well-being. These changes also aim to use public health capacity and capabilities to reignite the former synergies across key local government departments working to improve public health outcomes. They have brought about a fundamental change in the way that the public health workforce operates in England. The impact of these changes on the public health workforce will be charted in subsequent chapters of this book.

There is no consistent agreement on the precise competencies needed within the workforce and how they can be assured, the skill mix required for the future, and how the workforce should be grown and developed. Perceptions of what is needed have changed over time as the relative importance of some public health issues has receded and others have come to the fore. Nevertheless, there have been consistent groupings of the workforce around specific spheres of public health work, leading to the development of a specific competency to deliver health and public health outcomes.

Most public health professionals would recognise specialisms[4] within public health, such as the groupings of staff working in the areas of health protection (management of outbreaks of infectious diseases, surveillance of infectious diseases in the population, dealing with new infectious diseases), health improvement (promoting health, health education, prevention of ill-health), planning effective and safe services (on the basis of evidence of what works matched against identified

---

[3]   NHS Reorganisation Act 1973.
[4]   For a full description of settings for different public health specialist functions, see Griffiths et al (2005).

population needs), health intelligence (epidemiology of population health, surveillance of population health, ascertaining and assessing health need and health inequalities), and research and teaching in public health within academic institutions. Equally, epidemiology and statistics leading to an ability to assess population health status, health need and where to focus effort, as well as an ability to assess research evidence for its effectiveness, have formed, and still do form, the core of public health science. To these are now linked a suite of more managerial and leadership skills, such as project and programme leadership and management, effective communication and engagement, negotiating and influencing skills, and being able to work effectively with a range of partners and organisations.

The UK public health careers website[5] gives a broader description of the different functions of modern public health as follows:

Improving health

... working actively to improve people's health and wellbeing. This can involve working with individuals to give advice about healthy changes to their lifestyle (such as healthy eating or regular exercise) or with communities and the media to promote health campaigns (such as safer sex) or to advocate changes to public policy.

Protecting health

... promoting safety in the workplace (such as fire safety or the safe handling of goods) or the safety of the wider population (such as ensuring the safety of food, or protecting people from infectious diseases and environmental hazards, like noise, chemicals or radiation).

Maintaining and raising standards

... raising the standard of services provided to the public to help improve their health, and in making sure that public health is a safe and effective service. This might include developing specifications and setting priorities for others to provide particular services, as well as commissioning services.

---

[5] Available at: www.phorcast.org.uk (last accessed March 2014).

Working with information

... collecting, understanding, explaining, and communicating information about health. This information can be about the general health and wellbeing of the whole population, or about the health risks and health needs of a particular social group (such as an age group or an ethnic group).

Research and teaching

... investigating public health issues or teaching about public health. This can involve teaching about public health in a university or college, or setting up research projects to investigate specific public health issues (such as obesity, hospital cleanliness, climate change), and publishing the results.

Leading planning and management

... leading work to improve the health and wellbeing of the population, in developing initial policy, the strategies to put the plans into action, overseeing implementation and in measuring the impact that policies and strategies have on the quality of health and wellbeing services and the outcomes for individuals and communities.

The degree to which public health professionals will need skills to deliver the preceding functions depends upon where, in what field and at what level they are working. In addition, the ability to provide leadership on public health issues and to work in partnership with other professionals and organisations to deliver better public health outcomes are increasingly recognised as skills that are valuable for the public health workforce in all areas of work.

The agencies employing the public health workforce have changed frequently since the start of the health service in 1948 and particularly since 1974, as have the roles expected of public health professionals. England has attempted to take a more holistic approach to public health workforce development since the late 1990s. This has not been a straight line of development, however, being neither consistent nor constant. Much has depended upon government policies for the health service as a whole, the attitudes of those running national public health organisations and the changing views of the workforce itself. It is these developments that this book seeks to chart.

Developing the whole public health workforce

Public health has been a multidisciplinary endeavour from the early milestones in sanitary reform in the 19th century to the response to the Swine Flu pandemic in the 21st century. The specialist public health workforce was, however, historically dominated by medicine, with the remainder of the workforce in support roles, with little in the way of career structure, training or formal recognition of their professional experience. Postgraduate education in public health was restricted to medical graduates, as were the professional examinations of the Faculty of Community Medicine (later Public Health Medicine, and now Public Health).[6] The route to specialist jobs in public health was exclusively through registration with the General Medical Council (GMC) and via a formal training scheme in public health medicine, managed by deaneries, incorporating a series of service and academic placements and assessment via examinations and specific competencies. This route was only open to those who had undergone undergraduate medical training and had postgraduate experience of clinical practice.

The historic inequalities within the specialist public health profession were real but recognition of the need for change took a long time to materialise due, in many ways, to protectionism within the medical workforce around roles and responsibilities within public health. Community Physicians and Specialists in Community Medicine, as public health doctors became known after the 1974 NHS reorganisation, and their newly created Faculty of Community Medicine, became preoccupied with trying to gain standing within the wider medical profession, following their move from local authority employment (Lewis, 1987, 1991; Warren, 1997; Ashton, 1999). Although it was intended from the start that the Faculty would become a multidisciplinary body, its membership remained medical, with the exception of a scattering of senior 'honorary fellows',[7] due to fears that widening the membership would weaken even further what was

---

[6] The public health faculty of the Royal College of Physicians was established in 1972 as the Faculty of Community Medicine. It was renamed the Faculty of Public Health Medicine in 1989, and again as the Faculty of Public Health in 2003. It is the professional membership body responsible for standard-setting and overseeing training for specialist public health practice.

[7] This was a title given to senior professionals from outside the field who had made a significant contribution to public health.

already perceived to be a weak medical specialty. These attitudes were further ingrained with the experience of successive NHS restructures, where public health doctors were forced to compete for their own jobs.[8] Even when change appeared on the horizon with Acheson's (1988) review of the public health function, which acknowledged that the existing public health model needed greater multidisciplinary input, in practice, the report reinforced the notion that doctors should lead public health departments (Evans and Adams, 2007; Orme et al, 2007).

Change for specialists finally occurred in response to government policy in 1999 to create multidisciplinary specialists in public health posts. This has meant that, since the late 1990s, suitably qualified graduates in England from a wide range of backgrounds outside medicine have been eligible to train alongside doctors on the medical higher specialist training scheme for public health and thereby apply for posts at consultant status. This is a unique situation within both medical[9] and public health training. It has also formally brought a breadth of approaches and a range of backgrounds into the discipline of public health at senior levels – health economics, nursing, environmental health, pharmacy and health services management, to name a few.

Development of the rest of the public health workforce below consultant and specialist level came later. In 2001, the CMO for England identified three broad categories of those who contributed to the public health function (Donaldson, 2001). For the first time, this went beyond specialists to include the wider workforce, such as local government employees, teachers and voluntary and community sector organisations who have a role in improving health, although they may not always recognise it as such, and those public health practitioners working at operational delivery levels, such as health visitors or environmental health officers, who spend a large part of their time doing public health work.[10] Over subsequent years, particularly following government policy in 2004, which focused on changing lifestyle health behaviours to improve health outcomes, additional attention began to be paid to how to identify and formally encourage skills development and recognition for these groups.

---

[8] Crown, Witness Seminar 1, in Berridge et al (2006, p 57).

[9] The Royal College of Pathologists is the only other medical college that has fully accepted qualified professionals from outside medicine in its membership, but their training remains separate.

[10] For full details of the range of public health roles for practitioners and the wider workforce, see the UK Public Health Careers website, available at: www.phorcast. org.uk (last accessed March 2014).

In 2014, we are now at a point where: the majority of Consultant in Public Health roles, including Directors of Public Health, are no longer restricted to doctors; membership of the Faculty of Public Health is fully multidisciplinary; there is a formal, integrated public health training scheme open to all suitably qualified graduates; and there is an equivalent means of accreditation and voluntary regulation for individuals occupying those roles from backgrounds other than medicine to that offered by the GMC for public health doctors, and the General Dental Council (GDC) for public health dentists. There is also statutory registration for some public health practitioner disciplines and voluntary registration for others, and there are a number of schemes to skill up those in the wider workforce.

Discussions in workforce development tend to centre on competency, recognition and maintenance of competency as a way of assuring the provision of safe and quality services to the public and employers. Much of the debate about the public health workforce since the 1990s, therefore, has been about securing recognition and delivery of a quality service at all levels and including public health practitioners from a wide range of backgrounds.

At a time of further change for the specialist, practitioner and wider public health workforce following the implementation of the Coalition government reforms in April 2013, it is important to reflect on the developments that have brought us to this point, and the potential risks and opportunities presented for the future employment, development and training of the public health workforce as a whole.

The international dimension

The UK model of public health had long been admired by many other countries and it was common for public health practitioners to come to the UK to study, particularly the traditional public health discipline of communicable disease control/health protection. While the UK retained a predominantly medically led public health service until relatively recently, as will be discussed in detail in later chapters, some countries developed a multidisciplinary approach much earlier. In the US, for example, local public health officials have long come from disciplines other than medicine and medical practice, while the US Centers for Disease Control and Prevention (CDC) have always had a multidisciplinary workforce, although the leadership has tended to be medically qualified: today, the director and four out of the five deputy directors are physicians. US physicians have the opportunity to choose a residency programme – that is, specialist training – in public health and, in some schools, to enrol for a joint Doctor of Medicine/Masters in Public Health programme. While this comprehensive accredited training route is less well developed for non-medical aspiring public health specialists, there is a multitude of Masters in Public Health (MPH) options from which to select their preferred postgraduate course of study. The Institute of Medicine (IOM), recognising the need to strengthen the public health delivery system across the US, has published several reports on the public health workforce. As in the UK, the most senior spokesperson on matters concerning the health of the population is a doctor – in the US, the Surgeon General; in the UK, four CMOs (one for each of the four countries). In Australia, whose public health system was originally modelled on the UK model, the multidisciplinary public health workforce is well developed, although training programmes run in parallel for those from medical and non-medical backgrounds.

While the debate in the UK has long been about the composition of the workforce, in some countries, notably the US, there has been serious concern about the overall capacity of the public health workforce and a fear that it is inadequate. In the US, the IOM (1988) published a report, *The future of public health*, which addressed what were perceived to be major shortcomings in the public health system, including the workforce. It called for coherent workforce development and expansion, particularly to meet the needs of emerging public health problems. In 2001/02, the IOM revisited these issues through a multidisciplinary study committee, which published its findings in 2002 (IOM, 2002). In its report, the committee introduced a helpful new and broad definition of a public health professional: 'a person educated in public health or a related discipline who is employed to improve health through a population focus'. This definition took no regard of background discipline and depended upon all members of the workforce sharing a common framework for action and a common understanding of the interactions between the wider determinants of health, in short, an 'ecological model' of health. The report recommended collaboration between medical schools and other health education disciplines. It also emphasised the importance of health literacy across the population as a whole, which Derek Wanless (2002, 2004) paralleled in his reports to the UK government when he called for a 'fully engaged' scenario in describing the required degree of population engagement.

In 2007, the IOM published its report on *Training physicians for public health careers* (IOM, 2007), which recognised the need to retain medical skills within the multidisciplinary public health workforce. It set out the competencies required of doctors within that workforce, including doctors who practise in other fields of medicine, as well as those who specialise in public health practice. If we translate this across to the UK experience, the recommendations match the prevailing view in England that all medical staff are part of the wider, practitioner or specialist public health workforce and that any individual doctor may shift between these categories within the workforce during their career.

The US Association of Schools of Public Health (ASPH) noted in its report in 2008 (ASPH, 2008) that there were 50,000 fewer public health workers in 2000 than in 1980, so that fewer people were tasked with doing more for a bigger population. Further, they estimated that 23% of the public health professional workforce would retire by 2020, and called for more people to be trained in public health in order to fill the gap, and for federal (public) finding to support this goal. In particular, they called for increased emphasis on interdisciplinary training, to address, for example, the increasing prevalence of zoonotic diseases, as well as the social and economic complexity of many public health issues. The ASPH also sought to increase diversity within the public health workforce. Interestingly, their focus was not on the medical versus non-medical workforce, nor even about gender imbalance, but on increasing the proportion of highly specialised public health professionals from minority ethnic backgrounds, whom it was argued would be best placed to address health disparities within their own communities. This echoed the views expressed in a paper by Mitchell and Lassiter (2006) in the *American Journal of Public Health*, which asserted that only a culturally diverse workforce would ensure provision of culturally competent care, including public health interventions. As in the UK, the actual size of the public health workforce was not accurately known and so the ASPH's call to have a proper census of the workforce resonates with the ongoing debate about the numbers comprising the public health workforce in this country.

Looking globally at public health organisations, the Director General (DG) of the World Health Organisation (WHO) has, by convention, been medically qualified. The present DG, Margaret Chan, comes from a background of communicable disease control, bringing to the role a strong reputation of handling both SARS and avian influenza in her native Hong Kong. One of her most illustrious recent predecessors, the Norwegian Bro Harlem Brundtland, began her medical career in maternal and child health before discovering wider priorities in the environmental agenda and in public policy – to date, being the only WHO DG to become prime minister of their home country.

Outline of the book structure

This book charts the journey from a medically led public health workforce, with all those from other backgrounds contributing to public health outcomes confined to support roles, to one that is led by competent professionals from a whole range of backgrounds. Although this milestone has been recognised within the wider literature on the history of multidisciplinary public health and policy, the history of how it came to be and its impact upon specialist public health practice has not been written, a gap this study seeks to fill. Specific sections outline how the changes arose, what changes took place, what has been achieved and what has not been achieved, and discuss the implications of the next stage of development for all sectors of the public health workforce. Each chapter can be read independently. However, it also flows as a historical narrative, each subsequent chapter building on the one before.

The book starts its story in the early 1970s when medical public health moved formally into the health service structure. This is followed by: the rise of the movement for recognition of professionals from a range of backgrounds other than medicine during the 1980s and 1990s; the changes that took place from 1999, including regulation, training, competency and career development for public health specialists, and the position as at 2013. In each chapter, key government policies for health have been included to provide the backcloth to workforce changes. Each chapter starts with an introduction to the content. At the end of each chapter, key points are summarised. The position of the other three UK countries is reviewed in Chapter Nine. The book concludes with a reflection on what has been achieved and a discussion on how far England has come, outlining remaining issues.

The authors use the term 'multidisciplinary public health' to include all disciplines that contribute to the delivery of the public health function, including those from medical and non-medical backgrounds. The terms 'non-medic' and 'background other than medicine' have been used, where required or relevant, to distinguish those outside medicine from medically trained counterparts. 'Specialist in public health' refers to all those who are accredited and regulated at specialist level and are therefore eligible for Consultant in Public Health posts. A full glossary of terms is included in Appendix 2.

Whereas many of the changes that took place applied to the public health workforce across all four UK countries, the book concentrates on the England story as it is the largest country, the most complex and the one that has undergone most change.

In preparing the book, the authors had access to: archival documents; original research into the setting up of the multidisciplinary specialist training scheme (Wright, 2011); three Witness Seminars comprising public health and policy staff active during the 1980s–2000s (the first two held on 12 October 2004 and 7 November 2005, respectively, and both published in 2006;[11] the third held on 15 January 2013 and published in April 2013); published and grey literature; and interviews with some of the key protagonists and commentators from the time. All reasonable efforts have been made to check timelines for events referred to by interviewees and by those present at the three Witness Seminars.

Synopsis of book content

Chapter Two: Developing the specialty of public health, 1972–90

This chapter charts the early history of the public health workforce based in local government and the changes and impact following the move to the NHS of public health doctors and nurses from 1974. It sets out the struggles of public health doctors as they sought recognition from, and acceptance by, other medical colleagues. The section also outlines the other strong movements of the time: the rise of health promotion as a distinct force in public health and the development of a significant cadre in universities of non-medical public health academics.

Chapter Three: The multidisciplinary public health movement of the 1990s

This chapter charts how the momentum for recognition of public health practitioners from backgrounds other than medicine got under way and the start of change in formal processes to deliver non-medical specialist status. This is set in the context of key government policies that influenced change, which led to the opening up of opportunities for development.

---

[11] For the purposes of this book and to avoid confusion, quoted comments from the Witness Seminar held in 2004 will be referenced as Witness Seminar 1, and quoted comments from the Witness Seminar held in 2005 will be referenced as Witness Seminar 2.

Chapters Four, Five and Six: Changes for specialists

These three chapters centre on the changes for specialists from backgrounds other than medicine from the late 1990s and are presented as three discrete but interlocking parts of the story.

Chapter Four sets out the overall policy context and demand for public health skills as the backdrop for major change to senior-level appointments.

Chapter Five looks at the establishment of the new (voluntary) regulatory processes and registration for non-medical public health specialists.

Chapter Six ends the focus on public health specialists by exploring the setting up of unified training for both medics and non-medics to take them to specialist level.

Chapter Seven: The focus on practitioners and the wider workforce

This chapter outlines the start of voluntary regulation for the senior non-medical public health workforce working in defined areas of practice and the unregulated practitioner workforce. It addresses the context for meeting the development needs of practitioners and the wider workforce.

Chapter Eight: Where we are now? The new public health system in England from April 2013

This chapter outlines the changes to the public health and health care systems in England, implemented from 1 April 2013, and their rationale. It discusses their potential impact on the workforce and considers the new public health workforce strategy and what the future holds for multidisciplinary public health development stemming from this.

Chapter Nine: Experience across the other UK countries

This chapter looks at how the public health workforce is structured in the other UK countries – Wales, Scotland and Northern Ireland – and assesses how far each of the devolved administrations has progressed in introducing the changes to specialists and practitioners that have occurred in England since 1999.

Chapter Ten: Conclusion

The conclusion draws together threads and themes from previous chapters, summarising what has been achieved – as well as what has not been achieved – since the 1990s to develop the public health workforce in England. It sets the changes in an overall context by explaining why and how they happened and provides commentary from a range of public health professionals involved in the changes on the impact the English workforce model has had on population health. It concludes with a reflection on the potential next stages for public health development.

Appendices

Two appendices are included: Appendix 1 is a timeline of the key events in the transition of the public health workforce; and Appendix 2 is a glossary of terms used in the book.

TWO

Developing the specialty of public health, 1972–90

Introduction

This chapter sets the scene for later, important, developments in the multidisciplinary public health movement. The story starts in the early 1970s, when the public health system for England, which had been in existence since the introduction of the National Health Service (NHS) in 1948, was radically changed. Public health doctors, who had been employed within the local government structure since the 19th century, commonly heading large teams and with substantial responsibilities and budgets, were transferred in 1974 to the new health service structures. This chapter charts the development of this fledgling medical specialty within the NHS between 1970 and 1990 and outlines how insecurity and a desire for self-preservation among public health doctors contributed to a retention of a medically led public health model in the face of increasing opposition from public health professionals from backgrounds other than medicine who sought greater recognition of their roles.

This chapter outlines:

- the early history of the public health workforce based in local government;
- the changes and impact following the move of public health doctors to the NHS from 1974;
- the position of public health doctors in relation to their medical colleagues;
- the rise of the health promotion movement; and
- the development of a significant cadre of non-medical public health academics in universities.

The public health medical workforce and model for public health from 1948

Public health was a multidisciplinary endeavour from the mid-19th century but it was always medically led. Public health doctors worked within the local government structure: helping to implement major public health sanitation legislation for amenities such as clean water and battle infectious diseases; managing and leading the work of teams of public health nurses and sanitation engineers; and overseeing and running community health services.

Public health as a discipline for doctors was embedded into postgraduate medical training from this time through the Diploma in Public Health, a well-respected qualification offered by a number of UK institutions. The Local Government Act 1888 established the role of Medical Officer of Health in all provincial districts, creating a cadre of doctors with a licence to practise preventive rather than curative medicine (Berridge, 2007).[12]

Before the National Health Services Act 1946 provided, from 1948, access to health care free at the point of entry for all, a varied and mixed service model applied across the country; those who could afford it paid directly for care or took out health insurance. Specialist surgeons and physicians worked in some 1,000 voluntary hospitals and were paid with fees from private practice. Another 540 hospitals providing local care were run by local authorities with salaried medical staff. General practitioners (GPs) were single-handed, self-employed doctors receiving income from capitation fees from insured patients (Brown, 1970; Klein, 2006). Medical Officers of Health, as salaried doctors within the local government structure, held powerful positions, leading the teams of medical and nursing staff involved in the running of local hospital and community health and welfare services, as well as managing infection control and environmental health/sanitation issues.

The 1946 Act transferred the running of all hospitals to the newly formed NHS, which employed all hospital doctors.[13] GPs retained their status as independent contractors to the health service but were paid by the health service for the patients they had on their lists. Medical Officers of Health remained within the local government structure[14] but the sphere of their responsibilities, with the loss of hospital services, was curtailed. They were, nevertheless, still accountable for the delivery of a wide range of operational services, including child and school health services, ambulances, environmental health, the home help service, social work, homes for the elderly, and hostels and aftercare services for people who were mentally ill or had learning disabilities.

---

[12] There remained occupational insecurity, however, until the Local Government Act 1929 gave tenure for all Medical Officers of Health.

[13] Teaching hospitals remained outside the rest of the hospital structure overseen by Regional Health Boards, reporting directly to the Minister of Health (O'Hara, 2007).

[14] Some public health doctors, however, were employed within the management tiers of the new health service to assist with medical administration and planning.

The 1974 health service reorganisation

The reorganisation of social work services, stemming from the Seebohm Report of 1968 (Seebohm, 1968), spelt the end of local authority-delivered health care services. The review recommended the bringing together of the previous patchwork pattern of separate social services for children, adults with mental health problems and older people. The new social services departments were to encompass many of the services provided by local health authorities, including nurseries, home helps and mental health services. According to Webster (1996), this meant the death knell for the Medical Officer of Health role. A new role and place for public health doctors had to be found that would bring together managerial and wider medical and social responsibilities. The Hunter Committee, a working party set up by the Department of Health and Social Security to define this new medical discipline, produced its final report in May 1972 (DHSS, 1972b). Community medicine was born and its place within a reformed health service was established.

The 1974 health services reorganisation, as set out in the White Paper of 1972 (DHSS, 1972a), sought to further rationalise the health service structure in response to an ever-increasing health services budget and frustration at the continued separation of hospital, GP and local authority health services (Klein, 2006). All health services remaining in local authorities, along with the staff, moved to the health service. These staff included those in Medical Officer of Health and supporting medical administrative posts, health visitors, clinical medical officers running child health clinics, and staff running mental health and ambulance services. Social care, social work and environmental health services remained within the local authority remit. The post of Medical Officer of Health was abolished.

Creating a specialist identity within medicine and the National Health Service

Much thought and planning took place over establishing the role of community medicine within the new health system. The Royal Commission on Medical Education (known as the Todd Report), reporting in 1968 (Todd, 1968), had recommended the creation of a dedicated Faculty of Community Medicine, in response to recognition that there was 'gross deficiency in the educational and research capabilities in public health and those doing population medicine'.[15]

---

[15] Holland, Witness Seminar 1, in Berridge et al (2006, p 5).

This recommendation went on to expose a number of divisions within the public health workforce and delivery system, notably: (1) a major concern by doctors in public health practice that they would be seen to have a lower status than their colleagues in other branches of medicine; (2) a gulf between those involved in academic teaching and research, who included many eminent academics who were already Fellows of one of the parent Royal Colleges, and those in service posts; and (3) the decision to restrict membership of the new Faculty of Community Medicine to doctors.

The Hunter Committee (DHSS, 1972b) thrashed out the details for the new Faculty. Although the Society for Social Medicine (SSM), described as the 'powerhouse of non-medical input into public health education' (Berridge, 2007, p 405), had been established since 1956 and had, from the outset, a significant multidisciplinary membership, which included medicine, the non-medical voice was stifled by considerations of medical status and positioning when it came to its representation on the Hunter Working Party. Non-medically qualified academics in social medicine were overshadowed by the synergistic goals of the medical Royal Colleges and the physicians who had worked in the predominantly local government-based public health service – both wanting to see the creation of consultant status in preventive medicine. The desire of doctors working in this new NHS public health discipline to have parity with their senior colleagues in other branches of medicine far outweighed any serious consideration of opening membership of the new Faculty to people without a medical qualification.

The possibility of a subsequent, more open, approach to membership was not lost completely, however. The Working Party's final proposal for a new 'Faculty of Community Medicine' noted that: 'at a later date, and by agreement with the Royal Colleges, consideration would be given to the eligibility of non-medical colleagues practising, teaching or conducting research in the field of Community Medicine for membership of the Faculty' (Warren, 1997, p 45).

At the time, several of the 'founding fathers' of the Faculty were members of the SSM and one consideration had been that the new Faculty could be borne from a merger of the SSM with the Society of Medical Officers of Health. However, credibility for the profession appeared to lie with being attached to the Medical Royal Colleges. According to Smith:[16]

---

[16] Witness Seminar 1, in Berridge et al (2006, pp 66–7).

I remember the agonizing discussions that surrounded the foundation of the Faculty in the first place. Some people thought the simplest thing would be to amalgamate the existing Society of Medical Officers of Health with the Society for Social Medicine. That was ruled out by the main negotiators on the grounds that the Society for Social Medicine was heavily influenced by non-medical people.

As well as the debate occurring within the discipline, the views of three Royal Colleges had to be accommodated: those of the Physicians of London and Edinburgh and of the Joint Royal College of Physicians and Surgeons of Glasgow. Whatever the internal views within the discipline itself, achieving a proposal for a new Faculty that would be acceptable to all three Colleges was even more complex and required substantial compromise.[17]

During the gestation of the Faculty, it appears that little, if any, reference was made to a precedent that had been set by another Medical Royal College a decade earlier. The Royal College of Pathologists had become the first Royal College to broaden its membership, having welcomed in senior non-medically qualified professionals as early as 1962. The latter could sit College examinations, and were admitted as full members of the College, although the training and career structures of UK non-medical and medical pathologists were not, and have never been, unified.

Medical membership of the Faculty at its inception in 1972 was itself also a contentious matter, with many doctors holding clinical roles in community health being excluded as a result of the grandparenting arrangements put in place to control initial access to membership. These doctors worked primarily in the fields of child health, family planning and care of older people (aligned with social care). A minority had higher medical qualifications, such as a Royal College membership, or a higher degree. These doctors felt disenfranchised and excluded from their (former) close professional colleagues. Many of them subsequently found themselves accountable to a Faculty member (a community physician) in their new role within the NHS. For those community health doctors working with children, the report of the Court Committee into Child Health (1976) eventually recommended that Clinical Medical Officer functions should either become part of the paediatric workforce or should transfer into general practice, further reinforcing their separation from the community medicine

---

[17] Smith, Witness Seminar 1, in Berridge et al (2006, p 67).

workforce. These recommendations were largely implemented. This has been described passionately by Roden and Owen-Smith (2008).

Naming the Faculty of Community Medicine

The name of the Faculty of Community Medicine was reached only after much debate and deliberation (Lewis, 1986). A major issue was not only bringing together a diverse public health medical workforce from local government and administrative tiers of the health service, but differentiating public health doctors in their new roles from other medical practitioners. Alternative names such as 'Social Medicine' and 'Public Health' were considered, and rejected, by significant factions until, eventually, the compromise name of 'Community Medicine' was agreed. The biggest issue with the title of 'Community Medicine' finally settled upon was the potential for confusion[18] with community-based medical practice, in particular, general practice, and, as a result, some GPs remained antagonistic towards the name and, indeed, the new Faculty.

Berridge,[19] in her introduction to the Witness Seminar held in 2004, noted a particular irony in the choice of the Faculty's name. The term 'Community Medicine' was adopted just as medically qualified public health professionals severed their relationships with local communities as the specialty became part of the NHS and was no longer a central element of the local government infrastructure. With the 1974 reorganisation, their role was defined instead principally in relation to other medical specialties within the NHS.

From the outset, the Faculty of Community Medicine was a minor player in medical politics compared with the big and powerful medical Royal Colleges, both because of its newness and also its relatively small size. Equally, its members were doing work that was viewed as somewhat peripheral to the work of most doctors. Indeed, the fact that community physicians rarely treated patients set them aside from most of their colleagues in the medical profession. Public health doctors were perceived as having become 'remote' from the health of the public they served and were often viewed as health service managers rather than clinicians (Hunter et al, 2010, citing Berridge, 2007, p 406). The Hunter Working Party on Medical Administrators (DHSS, 1972b) had taken the view that community physicians were primarily medical administrators or managers, reinforcing this division from both their clinical medical colleagues and from staff working in front-line operational public

---

[18] Some people even thought that it was communist medicine (Griffiths, Witness Seminar 1, in Berridge et al, 2006, p 8).

[19] Witness Seminar 1, in Berridge et al (2006, p xxi).

health roles, such as public health nurses. Subsequent reorganisations saw the increasing identification of public health specialists with NHS managerial positions. As a profession, doctors in the UK have had uneasy relations with the NHS administration, a situation only relatively recently changing with the engagement of larger numbers of consultants and GPs in NHS management and leadership; therefore, to describe an entire NHS medical specialty as 'administration' in the 1970s was bound to have been a hindrance to the new specialty in developing its relationships within the medical profession.

The early years of the specialty of community medicine within the reformed health service

The NHS reorganisation of 1974 brought former local authority public health doctors into the NHS mainstream alongside those who had previously worked in hospital and medical administration.[20]

Each of the 90 new Area Health Authorities (coterminous with reformed local government) was required to appoint an Area Medical Officer (AMO) and designated Specialists in Community Medicine (including in child health, social services liaison, information and planning). Within each area, every district (a total of 200 across the country) had its own District Community Physician (DCP), with their own team of staff. Oversight of the new structure was through 14 new Regional Health Authorities. Senior public health posts at each of these three levels had medical titles and were therefore only open to medically qualified personnel. Terms of employment were 'equivalent' to clinical NHS medical consultants, but use of the title 'Consultant' by public health doctors was not permitted until 1988.[21] Community physicians at the local level had responsibility for assessing the health status and needs of the population within their area and were also involved in the planning (both service and capital) and evaluation of services. The AMOs, and, later, District Medical Officers (DMOs), had managerial, specialist and advisory responsibilities to health and local authorities and were involved in medical workforce planning (Wright et al, 2010).

The 1970s were a challenging time for this 'new' medical specialty. While the 1974 reorganisation was generally viewed by community

---

[20] They were joined by dentists working at the planning and administrative levels. The District Dental Officers took responsibility not only for managing school dental services, but also for advising the then Area Health Authorities on oral health improvement. District Dental Officers arose from the ranks of community dental officers providing community-based clinical dental services.

[21] Following the Acheson (1988) inquiry into public health medicine.

physicians as an opportunity to achieve parity with other medical specialties, all working together in the NHS, there were no objective standards applied to appointments and, anecdotally, it appears that the calibre of appointments to senior positions varied widely. Displaced public health doctors from local government found that they had to apply and compete for posts within the new health service administrative tiers at district and area level.

One former public health physician, later to become President of the Faculty of Public Health Medicine, commented that she was appointed to a specialist community medicine post immediately after completing the then two years' full-time Masters in Public Health course at the London School of Hygiene and Tropical Medicine (LSHTM).[22] She further observed that people who had come into NHS public health from local authorities were experienced in children's and social services work but were much less at ease with information and planning. Rivett[23] recalled that DCPs were:

> a wildly variable bunch of folks ... one guy who said it was not his view that he should be sweeping cholera from the streets of St Pancras; you also got the manager manqué and people who never succeeded in getting the time of day from the consultant staff.

John Ashton, President of the Faculty of Public Health from 2013, reflecting in 2004[24] on the calibre of people applying to enter public health training in London in the late 1970s, said that from more than 30 applications for a number of training places, 'most were thrown in the bin'. Rod Griffiths, another former President of the Faculty of Public Health Medicine, described his own experience of training in the West Midlands:

> I became a trainee of sorts in 1978. We trained ourselves. I got a District Community Physician (DCP) job in 1982. There were five districts in Birmingham; one had no Director of Public Health, one had someone who had the Faculty qualifications and the other two had DCPs who

---

[22] Personal communication, 2013.
[23] Witness Seminar 1, in Berridge et al (2006, p 7).
[24] Witness Seminar 1, in Berridge et al (2006, p 12).

didn't have the Faculty's qualifications,[25] one having failed Part I four times and the other having failed twice.[26]

Senior non-medical academics also had concerns. It did not feel right for them to be in the role of support staff to young and inexperienced public health doctors. As one commented,[27] although he was generally in favour of building up the discipline of community/public health medicine after the 1974 reorganisation, having public health as an exclusive discipline was 'bonkers'. He felt that the only way forward was to open up the Faculty to non-medics and to overcome 'the belief that having a medical qualification qualified people uniquely to do public health'.

Whether or not the 1974 reorganisation was good for the public's health is a much more contentious issue and difficult to define in retrospect. While the opportunity to influence the NHS was welcomed, the loss of the Medical Officer of Health and public health team from local government was seen by some as a great disadvantage in tackling the wider determinants of health (although local government retained responsibility for environmental health). Three former Faculty of Public Health Presidents (Griffiths et al, 2007) argued that the 1974 reorganisation fractured the relationship of specialists with those influencing the broader determinants of health. Hunter et al (2007) noted that, post-1974, insufficient attention was given to local social and environmental determinants of health by NHS-employed Specialists in Community Medicine.[28] Many became concerned with the planning and delivery of health services and accepted it as a price to be paid for securing a seat at the 'top table' when resources and priorities were decided. In fact, many DCPs, and later DMOs, retained a formal appointment in their local authority, as Medical Officers for Environmental Health (MOEHs). There were no resources attached to this appointment, however, and, in any case, the MOEH role related to Local Authority Proper Officer responsibilities for health protection, with accountability for dealing with communicable and

---

[25] Formal examinations introduced for public health doctors by the Faculty of Community Medicine from its inception in 1972. The Faculty later became renamed as the Faculty of Public Health Medicine in 1989.

[26] Witness Seminar 1, in Berridge et al (2006, p 7).

[27] Personal communication, 2012.

[28] A report from the Unit for the Study of Health Policy (1979) proposed the creation of consultant-level 'community health advisers' from backgrounds other than medicine, but the recommendation was not taken up at the time.

infectious disease outbreaks, and duties under Section 47 of the National Assistance Act 1948, but not for all the wider determinants of health.

The start of the health promotion movement and the Alma Ata Declaration

For many exponents of population health improvement, the 1970s were an exciting time. There was an emerging national and international energy surrounding the potential for health education and health promotion. Health promotion was beginning to emerge as a broader health discipline from the former health education, which had its roots in the local authority education service. Internationally, the Lalonde Report, published by the Canadian Government in 1974 (Lalonde, 1974), presented a new way of understanding health, proposing the 'health field concept' (see Figure 2.1), which largely rejected the dominance of the prevailing medical model of health. This concept was widely welcomed as a significant step towards an appreciation of the breadth of factors that determine health, of which health services or medical care represented but one factor. Lalonde was followed in 1978 by the global Declaration of Alma Ata (WHO, 1978),[29] which was central to the new way of thinking about and describing health.

Figure 2.1: The health field concept

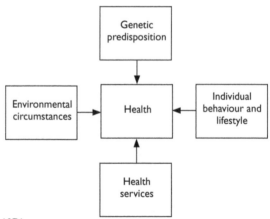

Source: Lalonde, 1974

---

[29] The Declaration of Alma-Ata was adopted at the International Conference on Primary Health Care (PHC), Almaty (formerly Alma-Ata), Kazakhstan, 6–12 September 1978. It expressed the need for urgent action by all governments, all health and development workers, and the world community to protect and promote the health of all people. It was the first international declaration underlining the importance of primary health care.

In the UK, the 'new public health' movement arose in support of implementing Alma Ata, including the development of two national pressure groups, the Public Health Alliance and its counterpart, the Association for Public Health,[30] both of which embraced the more 'social' or qualitative disciplines of community development and health education, as well as recognising the relevance of the more 'medical' or quantitative disciplines of epidemiology and health surveillance.

Within the NHS, in the early years after 1974, health education units were generally part of the NHS Community Medicine Departments, but in many, though not all, districts, they were small and under-resourced.

The 1980s and the beginnings of 'new' public health

Public health physicians in the early 1980s continued to be a very small group, somewhat marginalised within the medical profession and on the defensive. As Alwyn Smith, Faculty President during the 1980s, put it:[31]

> most doctors regard the practice of medicine as essentially concerned with the diagnosis and treatment of disease in individual patients and have difficulty in accepting that engagement in these practices in relation to populations is a comparable activity. The typical response to this latter marginalisation has been to assert strongly that public health is a branch of the practice of medicine and therefore essentially a practice mainly, and specially, for doctors.

One of the sternest critics of public health practice in the early 1980s was Sir Roy Griffiths, former managing director of Sainsbury's, who was brought in by the Thatcher government to review NHS management. His report, published in 1983, was scathing about management capability at the time (DHSS, 1983). This included public health doctors in their new roles, which, following the Hunter Report of 1972, Griffiths closely associated with administration.[32]

This perceived weakness allowed senior non-medical public health leaders to start to forge a way forward for themselves. As Goodwin pointed out:[33]

---

[30] Later to form the UK Public Health Association (UKPHA).
[31] Personal communication, 2013.
[32] Acheson, Witness Seminar 1, in Berridge et al (2006, p 23).
[33] Witness Seminar 1, in Berridge et al (2006, p 22).

the demise of public health physicians in the '80s gave strength to a non-medical, much more social model of public health development which was calling itself 'the new public health'. If public health physicians had not been as weak as they were the Public Health Alliance would not have had the impetus to start.

The Public Health Alliance, started in 1987, was multidisciplinary and was very much of the 'grass roots'. It attracted members from all areas of public health practice, including those physicians who would view themselves as progressive and inclusive. To others, the Alliance may have been a threat, as it promoted a vision of a different future for public health, based principally upon a social not a medical model of health. At the same time, academic departments of community medicine were recruiting increasing numbers of statisticians, sociologists and researchers from a range of social and psychological science backgrounds, and yet almost all academic departments were headed by doctors.

Health promotion and an emerging focus on health inequalities

The NHS of the 1980s became a difficult environment for public health physicians, who had worked in the service since 1974. Hunter et al (2007) described the role of Specialist in Community Medicine (SCM) as not sufficiently defined and many worked in isolation. The development of the 'new public health' movement of the mid-1980s in the UK was partly aimed at recreating links between environmental health and public health medicine. Ashton and Seymour (1988) saw health promotion as a means to achieve health for all, by enabling people to increase control over, and improve, their health and their impact on the environment. The Public Health Alliance produced a charter in 1987 which included environmental change in respect of some of the upstream determinants of health, notably, housing and food.

The Black Report (DHSS, 1980) on inequalities in health had been effectively ignored by the Thatcher government, to the dismay of many working in public health. Behind the scenes, however, many public health physicians were working closely with their local authorities – primarily those under Labour control who did engage with this agenda at that time – to introduce local initiatives to tackle health inequalities in the absence of national policy, which was to identify only the neutral term 'variations' in health, rather than the emotionally charged and judgemental 'inequalities'.[34]

Nevertheless, the 1980s saw the start of:

> a liberating and exciting time when the health promotion paradigm with its focus on empowerment and personal development began to challenge the dominant public health approach characterized by a patronising and patriarchal medical establishment. Rather than being based on a detached descriptive mind-set characterized by epidemiology, health promotion and the many hundreds of health promotion officers who were recruited and trained at that time were action oriented.... The flowering of health promotion in the UK began to create a reaction from within the public health establishment. They first attempted to encompass health promotion as a sub-discipline within public health.[35]

The health promotion community, however, favoured qualitative methodologies and was largely non-medical. Its tendency to see itself as separate from public health became divisive within the already small discipline of public health.

Internationally, Alma Ata was followed by the publication, in 1981, of WHO's declaration of *Health for all by the year 2000* (WHO, 1981). This emphasised the importance of inter-sectoral working towards improved public health, including the involvement of housing, transport, education and others. In the UK, the Faculty of Community Medicine embraced *Health for all*. The Ottawa Charter for health promotion was published by the World Health Organisation the following year (in 1986) and there was substantial domestic investment in health promotion programmes, in part at least as a result of recognition of the need for effective preventive programmes to address the rising tide of HIV and AIDS. In the 1980s, the Society of Health Education and Health Promotion Officers had at its height about 1,500 members, a substantial part of the public health workforce.[36]

---

[34] Bartley (1992) argues that public health took on inequalities as an issue because of its loss of power after reorganisation.

[35] French, Witness Seminar 1, in Berridge et al (2006, pp 36–7).

[36] French, Witness Seminar 1, in Berridge et al (2006, p 67).

The resurgence of public health medicine as a dominating force

The 1980s saw two major incidents that resulted in the identification of serious failings in the public health response: the outbreak of salmonella at Stanley Royd Hospital (DHSS, 1986) and a Legionella outbreak in Staffordshire. Sir Donald Acheson became England's Chief Medical Officer in 1983. He later admitted that infectious diseases had 'dominated my work'.[37] Following the two outbreaks, with the support of Norman Fowler, the Secretary of State for Health at the time, Acheson set up and chaired an inquiry into the function of public health medicine, which was published in 1988 (Acheson, 1988). The report made some ground-breaking recommendations, which were accepted by the government and implemented soon afterwards, following publication of the White Paper *Working for patients* in 1989 (DH, 1989). According to Acheson, reflecting in 2004,[38] 'Norman Fowler gave it political weight. What came out of the report was a small central unit to monitor health nationally and a Director of Public Health (DPH) in every district and region responsible for monitoring health.' Berridge[39] considered that the report helped to define the role of public health within the health service in relation to the new role of general manager announced in the earlier Griffiths Report in 1983 (DHSS, 1983). The DPH was to lead his/her team in the District Health Authority (DHA) public health department to: provide epidemiological advice to the District General Manager and DHA on setting priorities, planning of services and evaluation of outcomes; evaluate policy on prevention and health promotion; ensure surveillance of non-communicable disease; and act as chief medical adviser to the health authority (Wright et al, 2010). The DPH would be required to publish an independent annual report, very much along the lines of the annual reports of the former Medical Officers of Health, to publicly identify the main issues facing the health of the local population and how they should be addressed. The role of Consultant in Communicable Disease Control (CCDC) was also introduced to restore capacity and confidence in health protection.

Other recommendations in Acheson's report concerned increasing the number of funded places in specialist public health training in order to steadily increase capacity and capability nationally, identifying

---

[37] Witness Seminar 1, in Berridge et al (2006, p 18).

[38] Witness Seminar 1, in Berridge et al (2006, p 20).

[39] Introduction to Witness Seminar 1, in Berridge et al (2006, p xxii).

a minimum ratio of public health specialists to population,[40] and returning to the term 'public health' to replace 'community medicine' in describing the discipline.

While the Acheson Report did identify public health as a multidisciplinary endeavour, it nevertheless assumed medical leadership and support roles for those in disciplines other than medicine. For this reason, although it 'reasserted a positive role for the profession',[41] it was received with less than wholehearted support from some practitioners (Ashton and Seymour, 1988).

The Faculty of Community Medicine changes its name

In December 1989, in response to the publication of the Acheson Report the previous year, the Faculty of Community Medicine changed its name to the Faculty of Public Health Medicine. There was also discussion at the time within the Faculty about whether the word 'medicine' should be dropped. Many Faculty members in favour of multidisciplinary public health recognised that, post-Acheson, more of their close colleagues should be recognised as senior members of the same profession. But again, as in 1972, the Faculty's new name retained its medical orientation. The stage was set for the further challenges to come in the 1990s.

Where are we at the end of this chapter?

- Community medicine is now known across the UK as public health medicine.
- The Faculty of Community Medicine has been renamed the Faculty of Public Health Medicine.
- The Conservative government under Margaret Thatcher did not recognise health inequalities – only variations in health – but there is the start of a strong non-medical health promotion movement with these issues at its heart.
- The Acheson Report reinvigorated public health medicine as a discipline with a distinct role.

---

[40] A ratio of 15.8 consultants in public health medicine per million population (according to Griffiths [Witness Seminar 1, in Berridge et al (2006, p 24)], the precise basis for this ratio was never clear).

[41] Berridge, Introduction to Witness Seminar 1, in Berridge et al (2006, p xxii).

THREE

The multidisciplinary public health movement of the 1990s

Introduction

The 1990s, building on the changes under way for public health in the 1980s, saw the start of a concerted effort for more formal recognition of the role of non-medical public health professionals within the public health workforce, as well as increased opportunities for development. The aim of the gathering multidisciplinary movement was to challenge the 'glass ceiling' and to break the mould of a permanent 'support' role for anyone working in public health who was not medically qualified. This 'movement' was the fortuitous combination of: the growing evidence of the contribution made by non-medical public health practitioners in tackling public health challenges; a recognised need for a range of skills to tackle new public health issues following on from renewed health protection concerns and the rise of the health promotion movement of the 1980s; a group of people with dogged persistence; and a new, Labour government whose policy favoured a multidisciplinary public health approach to delivering better health outcomes.

What was new about the approach in the 1990s from the 1980s, however, was that the clamour for recognition was no longer confined to senior public health academics from backgrounds other than medicine, that is, university research and teaching staff, but included service public health staff in substantial numbers for the first time, for example those involved in the delivery of public health programmes on the ground, such as health promotion and health intelligence officers. The environment was ripe for change.

This chapter outlines:

- how the momentum for recognition of public health practitioners from backgrounds other than medicine got under way;
- the start of change in formal processes to deliver non-medical specialist status;
- the opening up of opportunities for development; and
- key government policies that influenced change.

Health service changes that had an impact on the public health workforce and the skills it needed

The National Health Service (NHS) and Community Care Act 1990 introduced an internal market with purchaser–provider contracts, general practice fund-holding and health service (hospital) trusts within the English health service from April 1991. This was a fundamental change in approach as District Health Authorities (DHAs), funded for the first time to support their residents wherever they were treated, changed into secondary care health service commissioners with accompanying population health responsibilities, playing to the strength of public health skills and methods. Family Health Service Authorities (FHSAs) were created to support independent contractors and the commissioning of primary care.

Further reorganisation came with the establishment, in 1994, of the NHS Management Executive,[42] whose headquarters were in Leeds. Under the Health Authorities Act 1995, the regional and district tiers of health authorities and FHSAs were replaced by 100 single – and powerful – health authorities, covering both primary and secondary care commissioning and contracting.

These health service structural changes had a major impact on the public health workforce and the role it played. First, they undermined confidence among the senior public health workforce. Almost all public health doctors at the local level were required to reapply for their jobs and/or compete with colleagues as the new structures started to take place. (As one interviewee put it, one day she would be interviewed by colleagues for specific posts, the next day she would be on the other side of the table interviewing them.[43]) Many senior people took early retirement, a pattern visible at each subsequent major health service reorganisation. According to Griffiths et al (2007, p 422):

> the standing of the profession was diminished in some eyes since it was clear that no clinical consultants would ever have been treated in this way. Unsurprisingly, morale was low ... the self confidence of those who remained was often undermined.

---

[42] The NHS Management Board was reorganised in 1989 into the NHS Policy Board and the NHS Management Executive. The latter moved to Leeds in 1994 and was abolished in 2000.

[43] Personal communication, 2013.

Griffiths et al spoke of doctors' anxiety about the possibility of competition from experienced people without medical degrees who could be employed to do the same jobs at a much lower salary.[44]

Second, the shape of service public health and the roles required of it were starting to change. There was an increased emphasis on improving health and a focus on prevention. The Conservative government in 1992 issued its strategic approach to improving the health of the population in *Health of the nation: a strategy for health in England* (DH, 1992). This was in response to the World Health Organisation's (WHO's) 'Health for all by the year 2000' initiative (WHO, 1981). Positively, this did indicate a shift towards a public health focus, though this was primarily through health promotion programmes and initiatives. It led to a renewed interest in public health and the wider public health role of health authorities, confirmed by the government's acknowledgement in the Health Authorities Act 1995 that a key function of health authorities was to improve the health of their population through direct purchasing of services or through influencing other organisations outside the health service. This was followed by policy encouragement for more formal partnership working between health and local authorities (councils), including the requirement to develop joint Health Improvement Plans (HImPs),[45] the joint finance initiative and the establishment of intermediate care and other collaborative schemes following the NHS and Community Care Act 1990.

The creation of increasingly large and powerful health authorities, overseeing general practitioner (GP) fund-holding and commissioning of all health care with (medical) Directors of Public Health (DsPH) on the board, supported by substantial teams,[46] gave a renewed impetus to the technical elements of the public health role. Public health doctors: developed the concept of, and then undertook, local

---

[44] This argument was to appear again in the run-up to the 2013 reforms, when a substantial part of the health service public health workforce transferred to local authority employment.

[45] The subsequent government under Labour responded to Acheson's (1998) *Independent inquiry into health inequalities* with its *Reducing health inequalities: an action plan* (Department of Health, 1999b). Their *NHS plan: a plan for investment: a plan for reform* (DH, 2000) set national inequalities targets for the first time. Local delivery was to be supported by HImPs jointly worked up between health authorities, local government and Local Strategic Partnerships, as outlined in *A new commitment to neighbourhood renewal: national strategy action plan* (Cabinet Office, report by the Social Exclusion Unit, January 2001).

[46] Acheson's (1998, p 31) report had recommended that DsPH should not work single-handedly and should have access to the advice of a team of at least two public health consultants.

population health needs assessments; advised on commissioning priorities based on evidence of effectiveness of clinical care; took part in contract negotiations with providers; provided analyses on patient access to health care; and reviewed the health impact of commissioning decisions. Dawson et al (1996), interviewing 10 DsPH between 1992 and 1993 about their perceptions of the job and the key elements of their role, found that they majored on strategic planning, networking, external liaison, motivating and organising their teams. In addition, since Acheson's (1988) report on *Public health in England*, DsPH have been required to produce an annual, independent report on the health status of their local populations.

There was interest in what the development of commissioning meant within the NHS for public health.[47] Some commentators reported on the difficulty for public health physicians in combining support for purchasing with retaining the role of independent advocates for population health. The Abrams Committee (DH, 1993), set up to review the public health responsibilities of the NHS as set out in the government circular to the health service, HC(88)64, concluded that it was the DPH who should be the focus for a comprehensive public health strategy, and who should fulfil such responsibilities as dialogue with providers, including clinicians, and overseeing the involvement of GPs. In many authorities, this propelled consultants in public health into prominent roles in support of purchasing, for which not all would have been fully prepared. These functions also meant increased managerial roles within health authorities, as Richardson et al (1994) found when they interviewed public health doctors and managers in two health regions in 1993 to discuss their views about the appropriate place of public health medicine within the new health system.

Many of the medical public health protagonists for multidisciplinary public health development talked of their experience within the large Regional and District Health Authority teams of the early 1990s, where they worked alongside – and came to recognise and respect – a range of contributory skills, such as health promotion, health protection and health intelligence, needed to deliver the public health function.[48] One former President of the Faculty of Public Health Medicine[49] (FPHM) said that, as DPH of a large health authority, she had a substantial budget that she could use flexibly to deliver her function and was able

---

[47]   Personal communication, 2013.

[48]   Personal communications, 2012, 2013.

[49]   The Faculty of Community Medicine was renamed as the Faculty of Public Health Medicine in 1989.

---

to employ any skills that she needed, such as a health economist: 'It never crossed my mind that the team should not be multidisciplinary'.[50]

This was at a time when good public health skills were in short supply. Smith and Davies (1997) surveyed Regional Directors of Public Health (RDsPH) and health authority DsPH in 1996 to ascertain the composition of their teams. Although distribution was uneven, they found that those delivering the public health function included pharmacists, nurses, research or information officers, and health promotion staff, as well as (medical) public health consultants.

Staff, apart from consultants, were confined to support roles in their teams, however. At the time, there was no expectation among senior medics that lead roles should be taken by staff other than doctors. One former RDPH,[51] reflecting on the 1990s, commented that as RDPH, he was concerned about filling medical public health consultant posts and having to take people who were more inexperienced than he would have liked, as well as fighting threats to reduce training posts. He felt that the prevailing view at the time was that although there should be more non-medically qualified public health people working in departments of public health, the idea they would actually hold DPH or Consultant in Public Health (CPH) posts and be equal competitors to doctors was regarded as something that was not likely to happen.

A commentator from 2005[52] pointed to the importance of the skill mix debates starting to take place during the 1990s in advancing the multidisciplinary public health cause. The public health doctor authors of *The nation's health: a strategy for the 1990s* (Smith et al, 1991) acknowledged that public health doctors could not manage this programme all on their own. Others started to grow an agenda on the back of this report.[53]

New skills and new approaches were needed. The move to commissioning, combined with closer scrutiny over what health care was purchased, contributed to the rise in the mid-1990s of the evidence-based medicine/health care movement and its widespread adoption by public health professionals. This followed the earlier research of Archie Cochrane (1972) into the impact and utilisation of health services in an environment where resources were limited (Berridge, 2005). The 1990s saw the start of the Oxford Centre for Evidence-based Medicine (Sackett et al, 1996), which led to the first Cochrane Centre being established in Oxford in 1992 and the

---

[50] Personal communication, 2013.
[51] Personal communication, 2012.
[52] S. Gray, Witness Seminar 2, in Evans and Knight (2006, p 71).
[53] I. Gray, Witness Seminar 2, in Evans and Knight (2006, p 17).

Cochrane Collaboration in 1993. There was also renewed interest in the mutual contributions and complementarity of skills of public health and primary care professionals in delivering population health at the local level. During the 1990s, for example, the FPHM had a Public Health and Primary Care Group, whose membership was mainly doctors who were dually qualified in general practice and public health medicine.

As the 1990s progressed, DsPH found it increasingly hard to balance the competing demands of paying attention to the wider determinants of health with contracting for health care, including contributing to unpopular commissioning decisions as health finances tightened. As Griffiths et al (2007) commented, this left many public health doctors being perceived by their clinical and other colleagues as mere administrators, siding with management and often responsible for rationing and refusing funding for new medical services. In some places, as the focus increasingly turned to commissioning rather than providing public health programmes, health promotion staff working on the delivery side were transferred to the emerging provider trusts. Once again, public health staff were tied to the 'vagaries of management structures for delivering health services' (Griffiths et al, 2007, p 422).

The health improvement and community development agenda

Following on from the developments in the 1980s, there was, nevertheless, increasing emphasis on community development and a growing interest in a broader approach to tackling public health issues. This was undertaken through focusing on the wider determinants of health and working with communities – 'professionals on tap rather than on top'.[54] There was interest in developing interdisciplinary approaches to tackling urban issues, under the 'Healthy Cities/Health for All' programmes.[55] As one former DPH interviewee said, each department in her authority had to have a plan of how they were going to achieve the *Health for all by the year 2000* (WHO, 1981) agenda.[56]

---

[54] Personal communication, 2013.
[55] *Health for all by the year 2000* (WHO, 1981), launched by the WHO.
[56] Personal communication, 2013.

Early changes within the Faculty of Public Health Medicine to create honorary members from backgrounds other than medicine

A key feature of the early 1990s was the preparedness of a series of presidents and senior personnel within the FPHM to promote the multidisciplinarity of the specialist workforce. As one former president commented, pretty well all the senior people in key roles at the FPHM would have had non-medics as part of their local, work-based teams. There was a 'frisson' at the FPHM about how they could be integrated in a sensible way.[57]

A senior officer from the FPHM[58] remembered multidisciplinary public health issues being discussed at FPHM meetings, including at board level, from 1990 onwards. There had been many earlier discussions over the years in the FPHM about whether there should be two or three categories of membership, for example, physicians and scientists, but that was deemed to be too divisive: 'There was this ambiguous clause in setting up of Faculty of Community Medicine in 1970s which said that at a later date there would be non-medical membership but that was well and truly buried'. He was not aware of the existence of this original document until well into the 1990s.

Following pressure from senior academics from backgrounds other than medicine in the 1980s – according to one academic,[59] 'there were clearly two levels of seniority but not of competence!' – in 1991, the FPHM created a category of 'honorary membership', open principally to those in senior research and academic public health from disciplines other than medicine. Some,[60] however, considered honorary membership merely a compromise, reflecting divided views on extending FPHM membership during the 1980s.

The standard for honorary membership was high, with publications being assessed and applicants expected to have at least 10 years' experience in a department of community medicine. It was the first attempt by the FPHM to widen membership. There was some ambiguity, however, about the status conferred by honorary membership. It was not truly 'honorary', as successful applicants had to pay an annual membership fee. It was not 'membership' in the sense that applicants were not initially allowed to vote or to be full members of the board (Griffiths et al, 2007). The latter changed when the Honorary Members

---

[57] Personal communication, 2013.
[58] Personal communication, 2013.
[59] McPherson, Witness Seminar 2, in Evans and Knight (2006, p 10).
[60] For example, Adams, Witness Seminar 2, in Evans and Knight (2006, p 62).

Committee was established, with, eventually, seats on the board and executive for the first chair and vice chair. There was some concern that it was merely 'token' recognition, as voiced by a senior academic: 'Quite a lot of people joined up – no vote or control, they just received stuff.'[61]

The start of multidisciplinary Masters in Public Health courses in response to demand from those not medically qualified

Request for support in development stemmed initially from multidisciplinary academic public health departments. A senior public health academic,[62] for example, talked of the 'mysterious' disappearance from time to time of public health doctors from his department of community medicine to annual conferences, from which non-medics were barred.

The creation of sizeable health authority multidisciplinary teams added pressure for access to development from service public health colleagues on a par with doctors. There was, however, a lack of a clear view of what development might lead to by way of formal career or workplace progress.

The establishment of the multidisciplinary Masters in Public Health at Cardiff University in 1990[63] presented a marked change in opportunities for formal development in public health skills. In 1992, the Masters in Public Health course at the London School of Hygiene and Tropical Medicine was opened to disciplines other than medicine. One of the first non-medical students, a former nurse, on the London School of Hygiene and Tropical Medicine Masters course recalled[64] how 'frightened' she felt initially to be studying alongside doctors. Prior to 1992, one non-medical public health practitioner did undertake the course but was not permitted to graduate with a Masters in Public Health qualification.[65]

The FPHM Diploma in Epidemiology became available from the early 1990s to candidates wider than just public health doctors but did not really aid career progression and was aimed largely at GPs. This was because, at the time, the only route to specialist registration, and thereby eligibility for consultant posts, was still via completion of the FPHM's Part I and Part II examinations followed by sign-off of a suite

---

[61] Personal communication, 2012.
[62] Personal communication, 2012.
[63] Witness Seminar 2, 'Chronology', in Evans and Knight (2006, p 91).
[64] Goodwin, Witness Seminar 2, in Evans and Knight (2006, p 14).
[65] Personal communication, 2012.

of public health competencies as part of the formal (medical) public health training scheme. One of first non-medical people to receive the Diploma worked in a senior health intelligence role at regional level in the early 1990s. She commented:[66] 'I think I was the eleventh person to get it and it very soon died a death because ... it was quite difficult to pass'. She then realised that she could not progress in her career on the back of it because she was still not eligible to take the next step in qualifications, which would have been Part I of the FPHM examinations. As she said:

> I couldn't join a training scheme, I couldn't get a consultant post and I thought this is ridiculous. I was working with medically qualified people who were pretending to be statisticians who patently weren't and I found it quite irritating.

She subsequently joined a group of people who had been brought into local public health departments in the region to prepare public health annual reports for the local DsPH. They petitioned the Regional Director of Public Health (RDPH) and the Regional Office to look at training, which, at the time, was only allowed for medics, and negotiated a diploma-type approach, people who could come in and do a mini training programme: 'It wasn't anywhere near the equivalent to the training programme[67] but it was a start.'

Mapping and gathering together the multidisciplinary public health workforce

It was pressure from non-medical staff in the West Midlands Region for access to development that led their RDPH, who was also Vice President of the FPHM at the time, to agree that they needed to find out who was in the multidisciplinary public health workforce. The resultant survey was carried out in 1994 and published in 1995 (Somervaille and Griffiths, 1995). It was undertaken under the auspices of the FPHM to establish how many individuals from backgrounds other than medicine were employed within the public health sector across the UK, what their skills were, what training they had received and how they had been supported in accessing training (Somervaille et al, 2007). A 'snowballing' methodology, starting with DsPH, was used

---

[66] Personal communication, 2011.

[67] Refers to the higher specialist training programme to qualify in public health, which was open only to doctors.

to 'find' people. One of the authors later stated:[68] 'the RDPH said it'll only be a couple of hundred people tops responding – we ended up getting a response of well over a thousand!'[69] Two thirds of the people who responded worked in service public health and one third were in academic public health roles. Of those in a public health role, some in senior positions, only half had ever received any training for that role, and of those that had, only half had received employer support (Somervaille and Griffiths, 1995).

The results of the survey galvanised those working in public health at a senior level to action. The RDPH commissioning the survey commented:

> We wrote to everybody we could think of asking if they knew anyone who fits this bill ... and a rolling sample emerged. We then thought we ought to get them together as their survey responses said they were without support. We contacted those who had replied and invited the first 150 that said yes to a conference in Birmingham.. ... At the second conference people decided ... they should set up a multidisciplinary public health forum and once that organization was created I stopped paying for the conferences. ... We also funded a booklet on what careers could be in public health.[70]

The presentation of these results, along with a review of career structures, accreditation, training and professional roles in public health, formed the basis for the first national conference for multidisciplinary public health held in Birmingham in 1995. Following this first conference, a small, core group of volunteers continued the mapping and fact-finding work until a second national conference was held in 1996, where, according to one attendee,[71] 'the strength of feeling was such' that the Multidisciplinary Public Health Forum (MDPHF) was launched. The conference determined that the Forum should be built around strong networks and that it should have a national coordinating group that should be set up for a time-limited period only. Groups were charged with reporting back to a national conference the following year. The multidisciplinary public health movement was under way.

---

[68] Personal communication, 2011.
[69] A total of 1,072 responses to 1,520 questionnaires.
[70] R. Griffiths, Witness Seminar 1, in Berridge et al (2006, pp 64-5).
[71] Personal communication, 2012.

The rise of the national Multidisciplinary Public Health Forum

The MDPHF relied on active people in each of the regions and UK countries to be its representatives. According to one of the core group members,[72] 'one of the founding principles for the MDPHF was that it was not to be a sustained organisation; it was a network of networks'. A local network lead from the South commented[73] on the gradual realisation among MDPHF members that ad hoc multidisciplinary public health networks were springing up in different areas. The one for the West Midlands, for example, met every two to three months and had over a 100 people in it.[74] The annual conference and programme of regional workshops gave networks a more formal structure. Following the first couple, the national conferences were funded and supported by a small number of the RDsPH. A business plan for the MDPHF was developed. A three-monthly newsletter started in 1997 as a way of communicating regularly with the MDPHF membership, promoting a shared endeavour to influence national policy and bringing about change for the workforce. Its circulation was in excess of 5,000.

The MDPHF, therefore, engaged with a wide range of public health professionals, many of whom had been largely invisible (Somervaille et al, 2007). Without this, the multidisciplinary voice of public health would have been largely an academic voice. The core group of the MDPHF considered that the health of the people of the UK was served best by public health professionals who were properly trained, accredited and developed, and wished to maintain and build upon the diversity of multidisciplinary public health to realise public health goals. The MDPHF's aim, therefore, was to ensure that the public health workforce was properly developed, accredited and regulated. It did not want to create a new and separate organisation to undertake these processes because this might lead to greater fragmentation. One of the core group later commented:[75]

> we wanted to pass the baton to other organisations to do that and talked to the Royal Institute for Public Health and Hygiene, the Chartered Institute of Environmental Health and the FPHM. The Forum was never intended to

---

[72] Personal communication, 2011.
[73] Cornish, Witness Seminar 2, in Evans and Knight (2006, p 11).
[74] Personal communication, 2012.
[75] Personal communication, 2011.

last beyond its usefulness. Indeed its main aim in life was to disappear!

The objectives of the MDPHF were to:

- improve skills to ensure that the health of the people of the UK is served by public health professionals who are properly trained, accredited and developed;
- maintain and build upon the diversity of approaches to realise public health goals;
- strengthen advocacy to promote the development of a unified voice for public health;
- promote the development of a single voice for public health professionals;
- address inequities in training and career opportunities for public health professionals; and
- work with relevant organisations (such as the NHS Executive, public sector organisations, professional and scientific organisations, and employers) to further these objectives (Cornish and Knight, 2000).

The Faculty of Public Health Medicine votes not to extend membership to those from backgrounds other than medicine

The spur to developing the MDPHF at the second national conference was the announcement by the President of the FPHM of the negative result of the 1996 survey of its members on widening membership. A majority had voted against opening the Part I examination to disciplines other than medicine.

One of the MDPHF core group reported:[76] 'June [Crown, FPHM President at the time] had to stand up in front of the whole conference and tell all the people in that conference who contributed to public health that they were not part of the family'. The then President herself stated:[77]

> the worst moment of my Presidency came near the beginning, when I had to announce the results of the Faculty ballot on widening membership to the MDPHF. I am still grateful to the many people at that meeting who understood my dilemma and treated me kindly!

---

[76] Personal communication, 2011.
[77] Witness Seminar 2, in Evans and Knight (2006, p 64).

She had earlier commented that:

> the [negative] vote resulted in dismay and hurt for many public health practitioners who not only felt disadvantaged financially and in career opportunities, but were also disappointed at what seemed a failure to recognise their scientific expertise and an unwillingness to accord them professional esteem. (June Crown, in Griffiths and Hunter, 1999, p 219)

As a result of this survey, the FPHM board decided that it was unwise to take a formal motion to its next Annual General Meeting (AGM) (Griffiths et al, 2007), where decisions required a 75% majority of those present. As one board member at the time reported:[78] 'to take a motion to the AGM which was defeated would have been worse than having no decision!'

There were mixed views generally within the FPHM and its membership during the early to mid-1990s about a move to multidisciplinarity. The Chief Executive Officer (CEO) at the time[79] considered that his appointment, as a non-medic, to the CEO role of the FPHM showed a commitment to multidisciplinary public health at a senior level after the vote. The views of sections of the membership were different, however. During 1995, the FPHM had organised its own workshops in different regions to seek views about widening membership. Those members consulted expressed a mixture of support and fear that widening membership would threaten medical jobs and career prospects for trainees, as well as reduce the status of public health compared with other clinical specialties.[80]

One former president felt that the health service reorganisation taking place at that time had much to do with the adverse ballot result.[81] There was a lack of self-confidence among public health consultants, especially those working in infectious diseases, who were worried about how they would fit into new structures. They felt that if non-medics became FPHM members, they would take their jobs and be cheaper:

> There was a feeling at the Faculty [FPHM] of real crisis – we were all going to be pushed out of the system – non-medics

---

[78] Personal communication, 2013.

[79] Scourfield, Witness Seminar 2, in Evans and Knight (2006, p 24).

[80] FPHM archives, 'Papers for the extraordinary meeting of the board', 29 June 1995, Box Reference 375789122.

[81] Personal communication, 2013.

were better at statistics and epidemiology and cheaper so they would not want us. It was a real question for the Faculty of where we were heading.[82]

This former president felt that this may have been a crisis in confidence related to the contribution of doctors to public health – agendas were moving towards tackling the social determinants of health, as well as improving health services – and may, in part, also have been related to the struggle that public health doctors had had during the 1980s to attain recognition alongside clinical colleagues, as outlined in Chapter Two. Long gone were the days of 'protection' and stability for public health doctors under the Medical Officer of Health in local government. Being a public health doctor in an ever-changing NHS was a quite different matter.

At one point, consultants in communicable disease control, who were more resistant to a possible move to multidisciplinarity than other public health consultant groups, threatened to leave the FPHM and join another part of the Royal College of Physicians (RCP) (Griffiths et al, 2007), fearing that the move to multidisciplinarity would upset the relationship between the FPHM and the RCP. More than one former president has confirmed, however, that the RCP was not disturbed about this issue at all – the Royal Colleges of Radiologists and Pathologists had both already admitted multidisciplinary members.

According to one former president,[83] the membership in Scotland was more resistant to multidisciplinary public health than in England. It was at this time, too, that honorary members of the FPHM, in frustration and irritation at the lack of progress, contemplated setting up a new body for public health practitioners from all professional backgrounds in competition with the FPHM (Griffiths et al, 2007) – a reflection of how bad feelings had got. The choice of change of name from 'Faculty of Community Medicine' to 'Faculty of Public Health Medicine' in 1989, voted on by members, had not helped the image in the eyes of non-medics.

The FPHM executive, therefore, felt that there needed to be a vote on this important matter because of the range of views – it had to be settled one way or another. At the time, however, there was insufficient support for change.

---

[82] Personal communication, 2013.
[83] Personal communication, 2013.

—

A changing climate: the Tripartite Group leading the multidisciplinary public health initiative

Undeterred, at the third national multidisciplinary public health conference in 1997 in Birmingham ('Multidisciplinary public health – what next?'), the MDPHF and Royal Institute of Public Health and Hygiene (RIPH)[84] issued a joint 'Statement of intent' for the development and accreditation of multidisciplinary public health professionals. The two organisations subsequently linked with the FPHM to form the Tripartite Group. The RIPH was included as an independent voice to balance discussions between the MDPHF and FPHM.[85] Each of the three constituent members was permitted two representatives on the Tripartite Group. The Department of Health (DH) was also represented. The Tripartite Group was also supported by an Advisory Group, chaired by the outgoing Chief Medical Officer (CMO), Sir Kenneth Calman, which brought in the disciplines of environmental health, nursing, health promotion, the Health Development Agency and the NHS Management Executive. A formal agreement across the Tripartite Group was produced in 1998, providing the project with a brief to create a national framework for accrediting qualifications, courses and the professional development of all public health practitioners.

The creation of the Tripartite Group and the national support it engendered was a seminal point, demonstrating a commitment from key national organisations to achieving professional recognition of public health professionals from backgrounds other than medicine.

New government, new initiatives

Despite the setback of the negative results from the FPHM survey in 1996 to widen membership, work to further the interests of the multidisciplinary public health workforce started to gain momentum, this time with support from the DH. Once again, a combination of circumstances and key protagonists supporting the movement enabled progress to be made.

The change of government in 1997 provided the backdrop for increased pressure to review and enhance development of the public

---

[84] Later that year to become the Royal Institute of Public Health by merging with the Society for Health, the latter mainly comprised of DsPH and a forerunner of the Association of DsPH, to work together on the development of a framework for education.

[85] Personal communication, 2013.

health workforce to enable it to deliver better health outcomes. New Labour expressed its commitment to tackling health inequalities and addressing wider determinants of health in its election manifesto and highlighted the need to stop the fragmentation of public health (Hunter et al, 2007). It appointed the first Minister for Public Health, Tessa Jowell, and started work on a health strategy aimed at breaking the cycle of ill health due to poverty and deprivation, published in 1998 as *Our healthier nation: a contract for health* (DH, 1998), which set health targets for the coming 10 years. The government also established an independent inquiry into inequalities in health chaired by a former CMO, which reported in 1998 (Acheson, 1998) and made 39 recommendations for tackling health inequalities, many of which required skills and capacity beyond the health service.

The DH started formally supporting small initiatives to investigate what was needed to further recognition of public health professionals from backgrounds other than medicine. It provided funding for a feasibility study into the case for national standards for specialist practice in public health (a study commissioned via the new NHS Executive Public Health Development Unit). A team from the London School of Hygiene and Tropical Medicine carried out a survey as part of the study between 1997 and 1999. According to one senior civil servant at the time,[86] the DH funded it:

> because a study saying it could be done looked like a way to make change happen and was a necessary first step to start to say to people OK, we can do this and there is a way to do this. If you say you wanted specialist standards sorted out this is an expensive business so you needed to show what they were going to do and whether it was feasible to do it. Do employers care, for example, and the people commissioning training because you need all of those people on board? What you can't do at DH is to march in and say there are a load of people who say they can do/are doing the same as doctors and want to be paid the same to do it. You have to find a way to systematise it and develop the argument as to why public health will be stronger and deliver better outcomes if it is multidisciplinary.

A report from the feasibility study was produced for the NHS Executive in 1999 (Lessof et al, 1999) and demonstrated the commitment to

---

[86] Personal communication, 2012.

develop national standards from both employers and employees within public health, a prerequisite before formal registration of specialists from backgrounds other than medicine could be established.[87] It thereby enabled the DH to approve a project plan detailing what might be needed to do the next piece of work of developing standards and how much this would cost. It also facilitated the allocation of funding to support the running costs of the Tripartite Group.

The second DH-sponsored initiative to start in 1997 was the CMO's project to review the public health function in England. This took a very wide view of the workforce – capacity, as well as capability – and included primary care. It operated through a series of workshops. Describing the project, one civil servant at the time[88] said that 'it was an organic piece of work – there wasn't a terribly set out recipe, it very much needed shaping. It went on a long time!' One of the organisers for the project[89] stated: 'it was really scoping out the whole range of what public health was doing and trying to achieve and what skills you needed'.

A report of the emerging findings (Calman, 1998) expressed commitment to developing multidisciplinary working. It explicitly called for different professional disciplines within public health to play 'a full part, up to and including the most senior levels' (p 6), and stated a need to develop career pathways, accreditation systems and equal opportunities for 'public health specialists from a variety of professional backgrounds' (p 1). The report was not issued without some opposition. One of the authors commented:[90]

> I remember, in the writing of it, it was quite difficult because I had DsPH ringing me up saying 'you can't lift the glass ceiling' and I remember feeling why not? But, at that point the Faculty of Public Health Medicine was supportive. The CMO was supportive. There were a lot of supportive RDsPH who helped push this through.

There were a number of other publications and reports produced in 1998 to continue the investigations into the status of training and development for non-medical public health professionals and to garner ideas of what was needed to improve the situation.[91] The

---

[87] Griffiths, Witness Seminar 2, in Evans and Knight (2006, p 37).
[88] Personal communication, 2012.
[89] Personal communication, 2012.
[90] Personal communication, 2012.
[91] See also Chapter Six on the development of the registrar training scheme.

MDPHF produced a 'position paper' on training, education and accreditation of multidisciplinary public health. A regional office-led Multidisciplinary Public Health Group produced a briefing paper for RDsPH on local initiatives for the development of public health professionals in disciplines outside of medicine (McErlain, 1998). There was also a follow-up to the 1994 mapping exercise (Somervaille and Griffiths, 1998), reporting on questionnaires from 532 individuals across the service and academic sectors. Most had had access to employer-supported development and training in the years since the first survey. A number of local training needs assessments were also undertaken. As one local lead commented, these were largely ad hoc.[92]

The Faculty of Public Health Medicine votes for first-stage acceptance of non-medics

Perhaps the most momentous change in terms of visible progress for the multidisciplinary public health movement came from within the FPHM in 1998, when the membership finally voted to open its Part I examination and, thereby, diplomate membership to disciplines other than medicine.[93] This encouraged the board to put a formal motion to its AGM in 1998, which, to the relief of the President, was approved without any significant opposition (Griffiths et al, 2007). By then, the Standing Orders had been changed so that decisions required only a simple majority (50%) rather than the previous 75%. A senior civil servant at the time[94] considered this a major factor in achieving a successful vote. She felt that the vote was actually quite brave of the FPHM, as she remembered lots of opposition from some of the medics. A number of non-medical interviewees referred also to a weekend meeting held at the time, when senior members of the MDPHF were asked to meet with key public health doctors in an attempt to persuade them that doctors were better at running things.

One senior honorary member of the FPHM said:[95]

> the pressure on the President from her peers/medical colleagues was tearing her apart. She was also getting

---

[92] Cornish, Witness Seminar 2, in Evans and Knight (2006, p 33).

[93] The proposal to open membership to non-medical colleagues on an equal basis was rejected and successful non-medical candidates could still not proceed to Part II examinations. Full membership of the FPHM was only achieved on successful completion of specialist training.

[94] Personal communication, 2012.

[95] Personal communication, 2012.

pressure from honorary members on an agenda she clearly had sympathy with. She managed to get it through. The successful vote happened then because of pressure from academics, the Honorary Members and the Tripartite Group.

The President at the time, herself an acknowledged supporter of multidisciplinary membership, said that she had also spent time over the previous two years setting up debates and doing what she could to prepare the ground while respecting the previous democratic vote.[96] She was also in regular discussions with the MDPHF.

Another former FPHM President,[97] however, felt that by the time of the successful FPHM vote, things were changing widely in public health and there was much more acceptance of what had been achieved by multidisciplinary public health practitioners through the work of the MDPHF. As he stated: 'the climate had changed and people recognised the contribution to public health from non-medical public health. The situation had calmed down. There was a general feeling the Faculty had got it wrong before'. One local public health practitioner agreed.[98] She attended regular regional public health network meetings that anyone working in public health locally could attend: 'there we were all standing in a great big room (that is medics and non-medics) with our plates of food and there was no distinction made between us'.

A further possible reason for the successful vote was that FPHM members felt threatened by the potential power of the MDPHF. It had, after all, identified over 1,000 non-medics and it could potentially have set up in competition as a voice for public health at a time when agendas were increasingly veering towards the social determinants of health and not medicine. The FPHM was in danger of being seen as insular and cut off from the rest of public health. According to a former FPHM President, it was better to have non-medics 'in the tent'.[99] Some influential RDsPH were also actively promoting multidisciplinary public health development in their regions. The RDPH in the West Midlands sponsored the conferences that set up the MDPHF. Others used the newly opened multidisciplinary Masters in Public Health to train their workforces, as happened in the North West.

The successful vote did not bring an end to the arguments between medical and non-medical public health over whether medicine should

[96] Personal communication, 2013.
[97] Personal communication, 2013.
[98] Goodwin, Witness Seminar 2, in Evans and Knight (2006, p 26).
[99] Personal communication, 2013.

be the dominant discipline. Lobbying continued, with non-medics arguing that many disciplines made up public health (McPherson, 2001) and failure to acknowledge this potentially meant that talented people would not join the public health workforce (McPherson, 1999). The medical lobby justified its hegemony by citing that corporate NHS boards would prefer to have a doctor rather than a non-medic on them (Taylor and Coyle, 2001).

Following the vote, there was an urgent need to consider what processes needed to be in place to take forward plans to achieve specialist status for public health professionals from backgrounds other than medicine – tackling training, registration, development and policy. There was a seminal meeting of the MDPHF and the FPHM President, where discussions were already beginning with the RIPH about establishing a professional register, and so, as one MDPHF member stated,[100] 'that was the start of saying "well we've got the Forum [MDPHF] and this network of networks, we've got the RIPH, we've got the FPHM, we've got the Tripartite Group"'. It was time to close the MDPHF down. By the end of the 1998, the foundations for creating specialists in public health from backgrounds other than medicine were ready to be put in place. Chapters Four, Five and Six outline these changes and assess their impact.

Where are we at the end of this section?

- Masters in Public Health courses have been opened up to public health practitioners from backgrounds other than medicine.
- The multidisciplinary public health workforce has been identified and its development needs surveyed.
- The FPHM has voted to open up its Part I examination to non-medics.
- The stage is set for the development of specialist registration for disciplines other than medicine.

Learning points

- A combination of policy-backing, senior people in influential positions in favour of change and a groundswell of bottom-up opinion can deliver change – right people, right place, right situation.
- Arguments for change were backed by survey support demonstrating the contribution made by a range of disciplines to public health.

---

[100] Personal communication, 2011.

- National public health organisations were prepared to work together to achieve multidisciplinary public health specialist status.
- Changes can be made with relatively modest amounts of funding.
- Public health medicine was still in a relatively weak position, subjected to organisational change while still emerging from its community medicine routes in the 1980s into a new policy world of purchaser–provider health care.

FOUR

Changes for specialists I: Setting up a multidisciplinary public health senior appointments process

Introduction

Following the progress made in the early to mid-1990s, the turn of the century saw significant changes for senior public health staff from backgrounds other than medicine. It had become clear that in order to achieve equivalence for applicants from backgrounds other than medicine or dentistry, certain processes needed to be in place for training, regulation and appointments at consultant level. These were given momentum by a new government with ambitions for public health and the workforce needed to deliver it. It is these processes which are outlined in the next three chapters, beginning in this chapter with an overview of the policy context and demand for public health skills as the backdrop for change to senior level appointments.

This chapter:

- outlines the stages in setting up multidisciplinary appointments at specialist level;
- outlines the development programmes in place for specialists from backgrounds other than medicine; and
- covers the move to a shared understanding of public health practice.

The incoming Labour's government's health strategy – creating specialists in public health from backgrounds other than medicine

The English White Paper *Saving lives: our healthier nation* was published in July 1999 (DH, 1999a). The focus was on tackling health inequalities by setting new national targets for cancer, coronary heart disease and stroke, accidents, and mental health. It also made, for the first time, a commitment to create a role of specialist in public health within the National Health Service (NHS): 'which will be of equivalent status in independent practice to medically qualified consultants in public health medicine and allow them to become Directors of Public Health' (DH, 1999a, s 11.25).

Other key measures from the White Paper affecting the public health workforce were: the establishment of the Health Development Agency (HDA) to replace the Health Education, to build and disseminate an evidence base for public health and share knowledge and good practice; a renewed emphasis on cross-sectoral and partnership-working; and the establishment of a public health observatory in each health region to identify and monitor local health needs and trends.[101]

The accompanying circular (DH, 1999b), issued on 6 July 1999,[102] instructed health and local authorities 'to ensure that the multi-disciplinary public health workforce has appropriate capacity and capabilities to deliver the health strategies'. Specific measures to develop the multi-professional public health workforce included a public health skills audit, creation of the new post of specialist in public health and a Public Health Development Fund to support implementation of the whole strategy.

The Chief Medical Officer (CMO) at the time commented[103] that when he came into post in January 1998, the Labour Party had already been in government for a year. The NHS Executive[104] was being disbanded and he took public health workforce development into his portfolio. He inherited his immediate predecessor's project to strengthen the public health function for which a report on emerging findings had already been produced (Calman, 1998). This project needed to be completed as the Green Paper *Our healthier nation* (DH, 1998) had already been issued and would be followed by a White Paper (DH, 1999a). He was able to include the sentence in the White Paper *Saving lives: our healthier nation* (DH, 1999a) that there would be a specialist in public health equivalent to consultant status. He later referred to it as 'an interesting process'. Labour ministers and their special advisers were heavily involved in policy development, and as CMO, he was responsible for drafting the White Paper with civil servants. There were

---

[101] The White Paper also included the production of a National Workforce Development Plan; although this was developed, it was never published.

[102] HSC 1999/152;LAC (99) 26.

[103] Personal communication, 2012.

[104] The NHS Executive was the management arm for the NHS. It was disbanded and its functions returned to the Department of Health.

a number of meetings with 'No 10' and Department of Health (DH) policy advisors. Ministers were primarily interested in the first part of the White Paper, setting health targets, and he was able to have a relatively free hand with the second part (as long as it did not cost too much money!), that is, the sections on public health infrastructure. These were changes that were important to the public health profession and for which he needed to get their buy-in – establishing the public health observatories and creating multidisciplinary public health specialists:

> I had to delegate the multidisciplinary public health initiative to the public health workforce team as I realised it would mean a lot of detailed work with the Faculty of Public Health Medicine and the General Medical Council (GMC). I felt the public health leadership would support the changes and, although some of the 'rank and file' might be less keen, with the force of the White Paper, a popular Government coming in and the appointment of a Minister for Public Heath there was enough then to charge down the barriers without the forces for reaction having any chance to fight back. So it was a tactical thing, a window of opportunity. There was a fair body of resistance among the Faculty membership but they would not be able to marshal forces against it with a Public Health Minister, Labour Government and President of the Faculty in favour it all seemed to fall into place.[105]

The Faculty of Public Health Medicine (FPHM) President at the time of the issue of the White Paper knew in advance of the statement about the creation of non-medical consultants but not that of non-medical Directors of Public Health (DsPH) – this was a last-minute decision. The CMO rang him the day before it was published to tell him. He was not surprised. There were good working relationships with the secretary of state and regular public health dinners with the President of the Royal College of Physicians (London), which, as an organisation, was keen to develop its wider public health role, 'So it was a *fait accompli* at that stage and no major backlash!'[106]

For others, the speed of the announcement about DsPH in the White Paper came as a surprise. A lead Tripartite Group participant, looking at what new national processes would be needed if there were to be

---

[105] Donaldson, personal communication, 2012.
[106] McEwen, personal communication, 2013.

specialists in public health from backgrounds other than medicine, including the legal aspects, saw the announcement and said to herself:

> stuff the legal bits, we'll just have it. It was just extraordinary and it was such an important thing for the White Paper to state. So we were going to have to go from a standing start to up and running in a couple of months![107]

Following the White Paper, national public health organisations, under the aegis of the Tripartite Group, and the DH were not slow to set in motion measures to implement the new policy. The DH funded the FPHM to lead a £60,000 12-month-long project to develop the role of public health specialist at consultant level.[108] Key elements of the work immediately following the *Saving lives* announcement included developing guidance for employers and setting up accompanying recruitment processes. Consultant-level public health posts began to be advertised by health authorities from 2000 to those from a multidisciplinary background with appropriate experience and knowledge, competing at open interviews with medically qualified public health doctors. It was notable, however, that the terms and conditions of posts for non-medically qualified applicants were often substantially inferior to those for medical consultants in the NHS, which were nationally agreed and routinely applied.

The success of the appointment of multidisciplinary specialists to consultant and, later, DPH posts was dependent on changes to FPHM processes and involved close engagement with senior honorary members. An FPHM Multidisciplinary Working Group was set up in 1999 and a revamped Honorary Members Committee was convened in September 2000, which later became the Specialist Development Committee. Membership included a non-medical honorary member representative from each English health region with a remit to work with the regional (medical) Faculty Advisers on drafting guidance for employers on appointments of specialists in public health, refining the specimen job description for consultants to make it suitable for specialists and acting as external assessors on appointment panels for consultant posts. In other words, the FPHM 'piggybacked' specialist appointments onto its existing (statutory) appointments processes

---

[107] Personal communication, 2011.

[108] Detailed work on DPH multidisciplinary appointment processes came later, in 2001, after the next set of health service reforms.

---

for medical consultants. According to the FPHM Chief Executive Officer:[109]

> we needed to ensure we had the same rigour for Advisory Appointments Committees[110] – but little authority to do this as specialists were not doctors and therefore there could be no requirement for a statutory appointments committee – we used (non-medical) regional specialist advisers to help.

There was continuing ministerial pressure for further change. Following a speech given at the London School of Economics by Health Secretary Alan Milburn in March 2000, which stated that it was Labour's intention to abandon the 'lazy thinking and occupational protectionism' in public health and 'take public health out of the ghetto' (Milburn, 2000), the FPHM held a postal ballot of their membership, which voted in favour of opening up the Part II examination to candidates from disciplines other than medicine. This was then confirmed at the Faculty's Annual General Meeting (AGM) in Scarborough in 2001. The FPHM President at the time[111] commented that the vote was 'really a turning point and I was very pleased – the most important aspect of my presidency'.

According to Somervaille et al (2007), the changing constituency of FPHM membership helped tip the balance in achieving a positive ballot outcome. The FPHM had already started to open up its honorary membership to a wider constituency by making the criteria less academically focused and enabling non-medical public health professionals who would be eligible to prepare for registration as a specialist to be included.[112] There was also an influx of non-medical candidates passing the Part I examination who were then offered diplomate status – and, with that, voting rights – within the FPHM.

The final multidisciplinary public health transformation of the FPHM came in 2003, when the FPHM changed its name to the Faculty of Public Health at the AGM on 24 June. The President at the time addressed the FPHM AGM in Southport with a banner behind her without the word medicine on it and then put the motion to drop

---

[109] Scourfield, Witness Seminar 2, in Evans and Knight (2006, p 41).

[110] The statutory process for the appointment of doctors to consultant posts.

[111] McEwen, personal communication, 2013.

[112] This process continued for a number of years until, as Griffiths et al (2007, p 423) state, 'the category of honorary membership by assessment was redundant and became discontinued' as all those subsequently registered with the UK Public Health Register automatically offered Fellowship with the FPHM (see section on registration).

'medicine' from the title to the board the next day, where it was passed. She regarded this as 'a big step – symbolic'.[113]

Shifting the balance of power – multidisciplinary Directors of Public Health

The next stage of Labour's health service reforms (*Shifting the balance of power within the NHS: securing delivery* [StBoP]; DH, 2001), while providing the new structure to deliver the 'NHS plan' (DH, 2000), which focused principally on setting up health service delivery centred around patients, improving quality of care and reducing waiting times, nevertheless gave added strategic impetus to the process of creating multidisciplinary DPH posts. The reforms replaced the 99 existing health authorities with 303 Primary Care Trusts (PCTs) as the local statutory health service commissioning bodies. This also effectively ended the previous government's GP fund-holding initiative. Overseeing PCTs, 28 Strategic Health Authorities (SHAs) were created as the statutory performance management and strategic planning entities. Two new national bodies, the National Institute for Clinical Excellence[114] (NICE) and the Healthcare Commission,[115] were also created at this time.

On 19 March 2001, the Select Committee on Health issued its Second Report on public health.[116] It had been set up to 'examine the co-ordination between central government, local government, health authorities and PCGs [Primary Care Commissioning Groups] /PCTs in promoting and delivering public health' (para 1). It emphasised the important role of primary care and, in particular, of GPs in the proposed reforms but suggested that further clarity was needed for respective public health roles across the different tiers of the new health system and requested that they should be properly resourced to take forward public health responsibilities. A particular concern was the 'vagueness' of the DPH remit and the lack of direct power associated with the role, stating 'the Directors of Public Health do not seem to us generally to be providing the necessary leadership in the public health field' (para 155). One witness, Jane Naish of the Royal College of Nursing (RCN), went so far as to state that 'public health is not particularly mainstream

---

[113] Griffiths, personal communication, 2013.

[114] Advising on cost and clinical effectiveness of health care treatments. Later renamed the National Institute for Health and Care Excellence.

[115] Monitoring standards in health care provision.

[116] Available at: www.publications.parliament.uk/pa/cm200001/cmselect/cmhealth/30/3002.htm (accessed December 2013).

in the NHS. It is not sexy, it is not high status' (para 204). The Select Committee on Health provided positive support for having joint DPH appointments between the health service and local government.[117] It also concluded that to bring about change, more emphasis needed to be devoted to the practice of public health: 'for too long the public health function has been dominated by a culture, mind-set and training scheme which stresses the epidemiology and science of public health' (para 242).

In the event, the initial guidance did not include the requirement for DPH posts at the local level. According to a senior civil servant working in public health development at the time, there were discussions among DH officials over whether every PCT needed to have a DPH.[118] The CMO at the time commented:[119]

> I was not consulted on public health issues by those writing the policy and I was worried they had not thought through the consequences. There was little consideration of public health in the White Paper and I had to get vocal about it. I was asked to put something in at the last minute. I emailed it and it was accepted.

Local public health posts and roles had, therefore, been preserved, with the intention to have a DPH for each PCT and SHA. The incoming FPHM President in 2001 had also become involved in the debate, the White Paper having been issued shortly after she was elected:

> I had to make a choice. StBoP was out and there was a question over whether there should be a DPH in every patch as the focal point to cover all the aspects of public health needed to deliver better outcomes to the population. I made a strategic decision to support local DsPH. I discussed it with the Regional Directors of Public Health (RDsPH) – I forced their hand as DsPH had to be multidisciplinary – I argued that medical [doctor] advice could come from health protection consultants so the DPH did not need to be medically qualified.[120]

---

[117] Formal joint appointments were introduced in 2006 following further NHS reforms.
[118] Personal communication, 2012.
[119] Donaldson, personal communication, 2012.
[120] Griffiths, personal communication, 2013.

The tactics worked. Lord Hunt of King's Heath, at the annual FPHM lecture at the Royal College of Physicians in November 2001 (Hunt, 2001), outlined the DH's expectations of what public health should do, the major task being to tackle health inequalities. He stated that: 'this generation of directors of public health will be from a variety of backgrounds not only medical. This reform offers an opportunity to make multidisciplinary public health a reality'. The intention was for DsPH to:

> assume a strategic role in coordinating a range of activities with a focus on addressing health inequalities. They are expected to lead in joint planning for health and social care services, to initiate and enter into collaborative agreements and partnerships with local government agencies ... and to foster effective community involvement, thereby bringing about the desired improvements in the health of their populations.

The move from 99 health authorities to 303 PCTs, each needing a DPH appointment, put pressure on existing medical public health capacity with the requisite leadership skills to fill all the posts. In particular, a number of DsPH from large health authorities were not interested in being DPH in a very small PCT and moved into other roles or left the service. Hence, the potential pool from which to fill these posts was depleted. When PCTs came into existence from April 2002, 216 DsPH had been appointed, of whom 38 were from backgrounds other than medicine (FPHM, 2002). The range of disciplines for the latter was impressive and included environmental health, nursing, health intelligence, health protection and health services management. The DH monitored the appointments. The distribution to DPH posts of those from backgrounds other than medicine was not uniform across the country. The North West stood out in appointing half of its 42 PCT DsPH from backgrounds other than medicine. According to the RDPH, he had a policy in the 1990s of sending public health practitioners from backgrounds other than medicine on Masters in Public Health courses, then creating pathways for their further development – one, for example, ran the Liverpool Observatory, the forerunner of the later Public Health Observatories established across the country from 2002.[121]

---

[121] Personal communication, 2013.

Inequalities between medically qualified and non-medically qualified consultants remained, however. Those from non-medical backgrounds were paid less than their medical counterparts.[122] Not all DPH appointments were open to non-medics. Each of the 28 SHAs also had a DPH lead. All appointments to these statutory medical posts were to medically qualified public health professionals.

The combination of many, some very small, PCTs (covering populations between 70,000 and 250,000), the costs of senior staff, and the depletion of capacity in public health at consultant level with the creation (and promotion) of many consultants into DPH positions (including some straight from the higher specialist training scheme) meant that, in some places, public health teams were small and DsPH worked virtually single-handedly. It was hard for them to combine a strategic with an operational delivery role. Many DsPH had small teams and a few had no staff directly accountable to them and so no one to delegate to (Brown et al, 2007). Some posts were never filled.

The setting up of a dedicated agency for health protection

There was concern about the arrangements for health protection following the proposed NHS changes. *Getting ahead of the curve: a strategy for combating infectious diseases including other aspects of health protection* was issued 10 January 2002 (DH, 2002b). The policy document raised the need to strengthen surveillance in the face of continuing and potential new infection threats,[123] as well as to ensure an integrated approach across all aspects of controlling infectious disease, chemical and radiation hazards once health authorities were disbanded. It recommended the setting up of a new national infection control and health protection agency, which would combine the Public Health Laboratory Service with three other national bodies (the National Radiological Protection Board, the Centre for Applied Microbiology and Research, and the National Focus for Chemical Incidents) into a local health protection service delivered by the new Agency, working with the NHS and local authorities to deliver specified functions relating to the prevention, investigation and control of infectious diseases as well as chemical and radiological hazards.

---

[122] Ashton, Witness Seminar 1, in Berridge et al (2006, p 61).

[123] National crises such as Bovine Spongiform Encephalopathy (BSE) and Variant Creutzfeld-Jacob Disease (vCJD), the rise of HIV and AIDS, foot and mouth outbreaks, and regular winter pressures, such as influenza and bronchitis.

In 2002, a number of medical public health consultants moved to the newly created Health Protection Agency (HPA), depleting further the available capacity for senior posts in PCTs. The HPA operated across England and Wales and brought together several former standalone entities, including: the Public Health Laboratory Service; the Centre for Applied Microbiology and Research; National Focus for Chemical Incidents; Regional Service Provider Units, which supported the management of chemical incidents; the National Poisons Information Service; and NHS public health staff responsible for the control of infectious disease, emergency planning and other health protection support.

The new HPA was established to provide expertise on potential health threats and took over much of the responsibility for health protection delivery. The PCT DPH still remained accountable for protecting the health of the population locally and for the provision of staff for on-call rotas. Arrangements between the two were via a Memorandum of Understanding (MoU), but it appears that there was frequently confusion over responsibilities for community control of communicable disease and non-infectious environmental hazards. There was also concern about the lack of a legal or statutory basis for the MoUs that had been created (Cosford et al, 2006; Hunter et al, 2007).

Categorising the public health workforce and refining the definition of competency: a key phase in public health development for specialists

The NHS reforms and changes to the specialist public health workforce brought forth a range of further developments – including setting up public health networks, moving to common terminology for public health practice and competency across the public health workforce, and developing programmes to support aspiring specialists to achieve the full suite of competencies required.

Formal categorisation of the workforce

The Select Committee on Health of 2001[124] had already queried the lengthy delay in publication of the final report from the CMO's project on strengthening the public health function, the emerging findings having been issued in 1998. The CMO, in giving evidence, said that

---

[124] Available at: www.publications.parliament.uk/pa/cm200001/cmselect/cmhealth/30/3002.htm (accessed December 2013).

the report was still 'with ministers' and the committee feared that the government's early enthusiasm for public health had been 'diverted' (Vol 1, para 46). Following this criticism, the *Report of the Chief Medical Officer's project to strengthen the public health function in England* (Donaldson, 2001) was eventually published[125] in February 2001 and confirmed the division of the public health workforce into three broad categories – consultant/specialist, practitioner and the wider workforce – and set the framework for development.[126] It gave official acknowledgement to the importance of wider public health for the first time.

The categories were:

1. The (so-called) wider workforce: 'most people, including managers have a role in health improvement and reducing inequalities although they may not have recognized this role' (p 6, para 2.8) (examples might be: teachers, social workers, voluntary sector staff, wider health care professionals).
2. Practitioners: 'a smaller number of professionals who spend a major part or all of their time in public health practice ... these professionals have knowledge and skills in depth for their specific areas' (p 7, para 2.8) (examples might be: health visitors, environmental health officers, community development workers).
3. Public health consultants and specialists: 'who work at a strategic senior management level or at a senior level of scientific expertise ... they will have a common core of knowledge, skills and experience' (p 7, para 2.8) (examples might be: consultants in public health, directors of public health, public health senior academics, consultants in communicable disease control).

Setting up networks

Following the structural reform of the NHS in 2002 and the creation of PCTs, there were fears about a lack of a critical mass in public health capacity. In order to maintain links and access to specific expertise across

---

[125] According to a senior civil servant at the time (personal communication, 2012), the findings from the project were fed into the 1999 *Saving lives* (DH, 1999a) White Paper and publication was delayed because the CMO 'did not want to trump the White Paper and work was in hand to implement this'.

[126] Cornish, Witness Seminar 2, in Evans and Knight (2006, p 44). The three categories arose from bottom-up working groups for the CMO project. For expansion of 'practitioners' and the 'wider workforce', see Chapter Seven.

a much more dispersed public health workforce, the establishment of public health networks was considered to be one way forward.

Lord Hunt's speech on public health to the FPHM on 13 November 2001 (Hunt, 2001) stated the following:

> PCTs will be the key foundation for public health but effective local public health action needs to be underpinned by a range of specialist expertise which cannot be provided in every PCT. That is why there will also be public health networks. Their purpose will be: to pool expertise and skills in specialist areas of public health which will be available to all PCTs; to share good practice and manage public health knowledge; to act as a source of learning and professional development. Networks will be flexible, responsive and evolve over time. They will not be an additional tier of NHS management or adhere to rigid geographical boundaries.

A *Statement on managed public health networks* had already been developed by the FPHM's Public Health and Primary Care Group and the Health Development Agency (HDA) at a consensus conference[127] hosted by the HDA in October 2001.[128] This was not proscriptive, but did emphasise that networks should embrace consultants and specialists, as well as practitioners, and called for agreed structures, funding, business plans and governance arrangements. In the event, according to Hunter et al (2007), central government provided no steer on how public health networks ought to be structured and there was considerable local interpretation of function, membership and objectives, although most operated at consultant/specialist level only. An exception was the London Public Health Network, which embraced membership from local government, academia and the NHS, and included people from diverse occupational backgrounds and expertise.

Annual conference for the whole of the public health workforce

Once the annual Multidisciplinary Public Health Forum (MDPHF)-led public health conference ceased after four years, the one place for the whole of the public health workforce to meet on a regular basis[129]

---

[127] Meeting whose intention is to produce statements that all those present can support.

[128] Personal archive of authors.

[129] The Faculty of Public Health (FPH) held an annual conference for its members only.

---

became the annual conference of the newly formed UK Public Health Association (UKPHA) in 2001. The UKPHA was formed from three pre-existing grass-roots/fringe organisations – the Public Health Alliance, the Association for Public Health and the Public Health Trust (the charitable arm of the UKPHA) – with the aim of uniting the public health movement in the UK (Hunter et al, 2007). It was used not only as a place to meet, but also for major announcements affecting the public health workforce. The RDsPH attended on a regular basis, as, frequently, did the CMO and other senior figures from public health.

Work on domains of public health and agreed competencies

The introduction of DsPH and specialists at consultant level in public health from backgrounds other than medicine also triggered a rapid need for the development of a set of agreed competencies spanning medics and non-medics. These would then both inform skills development and provide a common platform for assessment. According to a former president of the FPHM, working with the Association of Directors of Public Health, she had divided the overall public health function early on into three broad, overlapping domains or functions – health improvement, health protection, health services – with all three supported by public health intelligence and academic public health. This was in order to be able to capture simply the role of the DPH in the period following the latest NHS reforms.[130]

The other main initiative was to secure agreement across the national public health organisations and UK countries over what constituted public health practice – that is, to take the domains work further and develop specific statements on each area of practice. *The public health skills audit research report* of 2001 (Burke et al, 2001), undertaken by the HDA as part of the implementation of the 1999 White Paper (DH, 1999a), emphasised the importance to those who practised in all areas of public health of having skills in organisational development, partnership-working, leadership and change management to complement technical epidemiological and public health research-based knowledge and skills.

Ten key area statements of what constituted public health practice were finally agreed with the four UK country CMOs and were published in June 2002 by the FPHM and Skills for Health.

---

[130] Griffiths, personal communication, 2013.

Ten key areas of public health in 2002:[131]

1. Surveillance and assessment of the population's health and well-being.
2. Promoting and protecting the population's health and well-being.
3. Developing quality and risk management within an evaluative culture.
4. Collaborative working for health.
5. Developing health programmes and services and reducing inequalities.
6. Policy and strategy development and implementation.
7. Working with and for communities.
8. Strategic leadership for health.
9. Research and development.
10. Ethically managing self, people and resources.

According to a former FPH President, the key was to have a set of simple statements that all could buy into and that could be applied to training, development and revalidation for a multidisciplinary workforce.[132] The aim was to set explicit and achievable standards of practice. As chair of the Faculty of Public Health (FPH) Standards Committee she then adapted the GMC standards for ethical practice, at the time applying to all registered doctors, to provide an accompanying ethical framework that could be applied to public health specialist practice, both medical and non-medical. The 10 key areas were constructed from a shortlist of 17 areas, which had been themselves developed from a 'bottom–up' consultation at a series of workshops and in consultation with national organisations such as HealthWork UK.[133] Ten seemed a 'good number', so while some of the construction was a bit contorted, it 'brought everyone on board'.[134]

As President of the FPH, she was also discussing areas of specialisation and how to work with other public health professionals, such as those registered with the Royal College of Nursing and the health promotion workforce, and whether there could be commonly agreed standards across different public health groups. Hitherto, the only formal agreements of equivalence with a non–medical public health group were those that had taken place at the end of the 1990s with the General Dental Council over competency equivalence at specialist level between dental public health and public health medicine.

---

[131] See: http://webarchive.nationalarchives.gov.uk/+www.dh.gov.uk/en/publicationsandstatistics/ (accessed March 2014).

[132] Personal communication, 2013.

[133] HealthWork UK, the Sector Skills Council responsible for health, was later renamed Skills for Health.

[134] Griffiths, personal communication, 2013.

Following the issue of the 10 key area statements on public health, HealthWork UK was commissioned by the DH, as part of the implementation of the *Saving lives* White Paper (DH, 1999a), to work with national public health organisations and the workforce to develop detailed national occupational standards for public health practice. The project was jointly funded by the Qualifications and Curriculum Authority and the UK Health Departments. Skills for Health (formerly HealthWork UK) published their *National Occupational Standards for Public Health* in 2004. Also in that year, the new Nursing and Midwifery Council (which replaced the UK Central Council for Nursing as the sole statutory regulator of nurses and midwives in the UK) launched its standards of proficiency for specialist community public health nurses as part of its new statutory register.

'Top-up' development for aspiring specialists

By 2002, the appointment of a number of specialists and DsPH from backgrounds other than medicine highlighted the need for some competency development, particularly if these new non-medical public health specialists were to be formally regulated and meet the required standards.[135]

As part of the process of setting up regulatory measures for these new specialists in public health, the Public Health Resource Unit (PHRU) was commissioned to develop a competency framework suitable for retrospective assessment of specialists for registration. In undertaking this work, the PHRU identified a local 'top-up' need for development of those specialists who would be preparing portfolios of work to meet set standards.[136] On self-assessment, most aspiring specialists identified at least one competency gap, which was unsurprising as specialists had not hitherto had access to formal training schemes. This was then taken up nationally through the DH public health development group. The DH allocated approximate £800,000 over a two-year period to public health development: 'It helped get things going on the group at local level'.[137] It funded some of the early public health

---

[135] Once the UK Public Health Register was launched in 2003, non-medical DsPH were given provisional registration pending completion of a satisfactory portfolio to meet standards. This was for reasons of public protection.

[136] Proposal from the PHRU for funding, 2002; Development Needs Assessment Centre report, January to December 2003, PHRU. Both in personal archive of the authors.

[137] Personal communication, 2012.

training schemes set up in the Postgraduate Deaneries[138] and public health leadership schemes (London and West Midlands), which were multidisciplinary, that is, open to senior public health professionals from a range of backgrounds, including medicine, as well as multi-agency participants, including health and local government. Individual regions decided independently how they wished to spend their development fund allocation.

The DH also funded the PHRU to run a time-limited Development Needs Assessment Centre (DNAC) to make available to each region consultant-level expertise to support portfolio preparation for application for retrospective recognition by the newly created UK Public Health Register (UKPHR) as a specialist.[139] The resource helped regional teams set up workshops to explain registration routes, provided criteria in assessing potential applicants, supplied people to sit on local panels to consider applicants for top-up training schemes, trained local support teams, contributed to local events identifying competency gaps and supported those building portfolios.[140] Support was offered to those seeking specialist status, as well as to non-medical DsPH, who now needed to achieve registration with the UKPHR.

Moves to increase public health capacity

By the start of 2004, there were serious concerns across England about public health capacity at a senior enough level, despite the development of specialists under way across the country. Derek Wanless, commissioned by Her Majesty's Treasury, reported in 2002 and, again, in 2004 (Wanless, 2002, 2004) on the challenge of having an affordable health service without a wholesale population shift in attitude to health. He criticised the lack of a public health strategy, insufficient leadership and a public health workforce not fit for purpose. He called for a refocus of public health energy from the NHS being a sickness service towards a service that addressed key lifestyle and environmental risks.

The joint response to the 2002 Wanless Report from the Faculty of Public Health (FPH), the Local Government Association (LGA),

---

[138] Organisations responsible for postgraduate medical and dental education and training.

[139] The scheme ran for three years to match the three-year window for aspiring specialists to submit retrospective portfolios (see Chapter Five).

[140] DNAC report, January to December 2003, PHRU; personal archive of the authors. The schemes could not be called fast-track schemes as registrars on the training scheme considered that non-medical specialists would be reaching consultant status by an easier backdoor route. Witness Seminar 2, in Evans and Knight (2006, p 45).

NHS Confederation, UKPHA and Association of Public Health Observatories (APHO) on 14 November 2003[141] supported the need to mainstream public health when it stated: 'public health is not the prerogative of the NHS or indeed any single part of the public sector. It is an intrinsic part of the mainstream activities of both the statutory and non-statutory sectors'.

The FPH had been concerned for a while about having sufficient senior-level capacity to meet all the requirements of the reconfigured health service. It organised a series of surveys and of workshops around the country to get some 'bottom-up' feedback on how to increase capacity quickly. Suggestions included: not having single-handed DsPH in PCTs; doing more to work jointly with primary care professionals such as General Practitioners (GPs) and health visitors; and looking imaginatively at different ways of mobilising capacity by accessing other relevant workforces, such as those within local government. The FPH was also undertaking annual surveys (funded by the DH) of the specialist public health workforce in the UK. The 2003 survey formerly reported in March 2004 to the FPH board.[142] This identified shortfalls in senior public health capacity in PCTs, as well as in health protection and academic public health. If the FPH aspirational target of 2.5 whole-time equivalent (wte) consultants and specialists per 100,000 population was to be met, an increase in capacity of 40% would be needed. The overall level of total specialist public health capacity fell from 22.2 per million population in the 2003 report to 18.5 per million population in the 2005 survey report.[143] Although UKPHR had opened in mid-2003, specialists from backgrounds other than medicine did not start to achieve registration in significant numbers to help fill this gap until 2005/06 – this brought a total additional capacity of 400.

These concerns about both capacity and capability of the public health workforce to deliver change were given further impetus as the profile of the public health workforce gained new prominence following new policy and structural health service changes in England in 2005 and 2006.

The *Choosing health* White Paper (DH, 2004b) – the government's unstated but apparent response to the two Wanless Reports – focused on six themes as ways to reduce health inequalities: sexual health, mental health, obesity, smoking reduction, reduction in alcohol intake and increasing exercise. It promoted a personalisation agenda backed

---

[141] 'Statement from the FPH, NHS Confederation, LGA, APHO, UKPHA, 14 November 2003'; personal archive of the authors.

[142] Paper by Perlman and Gray. Personal archive of the authors.

[143] Paper by Gray and Sandberg. Personal archive of the authors.

by informed choice for the public, whereby individuals would be empowered to make healthy lifestyle choices. It also signalled, for the first time, a commitment to developing the whole of the public health workforce – consultants and specialists in leadership and strategic roles – but also accessing a whole range of other relevant skills targeted at health improvement, including pharmacists and dentists. The new role of 'health trainers' recruited from local communities and trained to uniform standards was introduced with pump-priming funding from the DH. Implementation of the whole of the White Paper was backed by DH funding to PCTs. As one interviewee stated, the 'fully engaged scenario', as outlined by Wanless, was attractive to the government as it promised potential cost savings from NHS provision by moving 'upstream'.[144]

At the same time, a long-term project led by the DH to bring the whole of the NHS workforce (with the exception of doctors, dentists and very senior managers) into a single pay framework called Agenda for Change (AfC) started to be implemented from 2004 (DH, 2004c).[145] This divided the workforce into 12 pay bands and produced profiles for different health professionals. The initiative was to prove crucial to enabling specialists in public health to approach equivalence in pay with public health doctors, which had been a bone of contention since the introduction of specialists in public health. Wright (2007) argues that while not specifically aimed at the public health workforce, AfC did have the result of leading to a coherent approach to job definitions and pay scales in the NHS for public health for the first time. Prior to this, PCTs could advertise posts with the title of specialist in public health at any salary, and often at much lower pay than the nationally agreed rate for medically qualified consultants. For public health, therefore, AfC provided coordination of appropriate pay with appropriate competencies for specified roles.

The DH funded a specific initiative in 2005 to develop a suite of job profiles at different AfC bands in the workforce for public health. These not only related to specialists, but also, among others, to those working in health promotion and health intelligence. Moreover under AfC, the medical public health consultant-equivalent profile and pay grade (8d or 9[146]) was given the title of 'consultant' to replace that of 'specialist', which had been in common use for non-medics

---

[144] Personal communication, 2013.

[145] See also: http://www.nhsemployers.org/PayAndContracts/AgendaForChange/ Pages/Afc-Homepage.aspx (accessed February 2014).

[146] AfC bands span 1–9, with band 8 split into four (8a–d), that is, 12 levels in total.

—

beforehand.[147] Confirmation of the title 'consultant in public health' was not met with universal support from public health doctors, a number of whom chose to retain the title of 'consultant in public health *medicine*' to differentiate themselves from non-medical specialists. Following the publication of AfC bandings, consultant in public health posts were advertised, for non-medical applicants, at bands 8d or 9.

Further reorganisation

The perceived failure of small PCTs to deliver on commissioning, together with perceived opportunities for management savings, led to further health service restructuring by reducing, through mergers, the number of PCTs from 303 to 152 and the number of SHAs from 28 to 10, with effect from April 2006 (DH, 2005). As a result PCT-resident populations from April 2006 increased to between about 250,000 and 1 million and boundaries became more often coterminous with (upper-tier[148]) local authorities.[149]

The changes meant, once again, that many consultants needed to apply for their posts in the new structures. There were initial concerns from the British Medical Association (BMA) about a forced reduction in consultant public health capacity from merged PCTs (BMA Parliamentary Unit, 2011).

The FPH undertook a displacement survey in January 2007[150] to investigate likely losses as a result of organisational change. Of the 342 respondents, it found that two thirds were in PCTs that were reconfiguring, and in half of the latter, consultants reported having to apply for their own job in the new structure. The bulk expected to still have a public health job in the NHS following reorganisation. An analysis of the health service workforce from the Information Centre for Health and Social Care collection based on 81% of AfC returns[151] found 400 staff at the senior level on band 8d and around 800 on bands 8a–c. A breakdown of the total workforce (ie all AfC bands 1–9) found nearly half working in health promotion and a quarter in health protection. Only 75 were in health intelligence posts. Further attempts

---

[147] This was because specialist nurses were on lower AfC gradings and there was already a precedent at the senior grade for use of the title 'consultant' by clinical psychologists.

[148] County council, metropolitan or unitary authorities.

[149] Populations were smaller in some London and other coterminous PCTs.

[150] Personal archive of the authors.

[151] Duggan, A., Bourne, A. and Gibson, S. (April 2007) unpublished report from Information Centre for Health and Social Care, FPH archives.

were made to capture more accurately the public health workforce through electronic staff records and to establish a minimum data set for public health, but without success.[152]

The 2006 reforms were important, however, in raising the profile of public health in two particular aspects. First, introducing an expectation of formal joint appointments of health service PCT DsPH with partner local authorities shifted the focus of service public health towards health improvement. Second, to boost performance, the introduction of *World class commissioning* competencies (DH, 2007) by the DH in December 2007,[153] and assessment of PCTs against them, gave prominence to key public health activities within the health service at the time, such as assessment of health need, working with patients and the public, and assessment of the clinical and cost-effectiveness of services that were commissioned. In the annual NHS operating framework for 2007/08,[154] there was increased emphasis on operational performance indicators (so-called 'vital signs') for PCTs, covering public health issues such as smoking, vaccination rates, breastfeeding and obesity (DH, 2006). So, PCTs would now be held to account for achievement of public health goals.

Formal partnerships with local authorities – public health begins its return to local government

The government further encouraged the setting up of joint DPH appointments between PCTs and local authorities by increasing joint accountability through three-year Local Area Agreements between local and central government. These built on previous multi-agency Local Strategic Partnerships and set targets to improve health outcomes, which were to be informed by new Joint Strategic Needs Assessments (covering local authority and health interests), Comprehensive Area Agreements and the setting of joint targets within Public Sector Agreements (PSAs) (DH, 2005). A new framework was emerging that emphasised a whole systems approach based upon the importance of partnership-working across the NHS, local government and the third (voluntary) sector (Hannaway et al, 2007).

The specimen job description for the role of DPH, updated by the FPH in response to the changes, emphasised its major role in

---

[152] Minutes from national workshop hosted by the DH, 18 September 2008. Personal archive of the authors.

[153] The DH issued its vision and competency framework in December 2007 for the way health and care services should be commissioned.

[154] Second operating framework issued by the DH for the NHS.

---

strategic leadership, as well as unique oversight of the three domains that contributed to enhancing population health within their field of influence (health improvement, health protection and health and social care quality). The reduction in the number of PCTs made it easier for DsPH to (re)build substantial public health teams and to recreate the senior posts of Deputy and Assistant DPH for larger PCTs. By 2010, it has been estimated that over 80% of DPH appointments in England were joint appointments between the NHS and local government (Maryon-Davis, 2010). One interviewee commented, however, that 'it was clear that some were joint in name only with life going on much as before!'[155] Importantly, many joint DPH posts remained fully funded by the NHS until March 2013.

As far as local authorities were concerned, the picture was mixed – anecdotally at least, as there was a scarcity of objective research. Some were keen to appoint a doctor to the position of DPH, while others were delighted at the prospect of being liberated from the requirement to appoint a doctor to this position.

The increased prominence of the DPH and public health role within PCTs was not without its problems, however. Pittam and Wright (2011) talk of 'role creep' for DsPH, resulting from repeated reorganisations and how the rapid increase in the role's strategic importance challenged the specialist training programme to keep abreast. Concerns were also being raised about how the 'traditional' independence of the role could be maintained in the face of corporate responsibility at a time of cutbacks. DsPH were also faced with the complexities and challenges of balancing accountabilities across the secretary of state for health, local council, NHS and public health teams. These concerns were to re-emerge in the run-up to the 2013 reforms.

Academic public health

There were continuing concerns about a decline in academic public health capacity during the early 2000s, as well as widening gaps between service and academic public health (Dunkley and Wright, 2010). The public health workforce on the ground needed access to the best evidence relevant to issues they were facing if change was to take place in health outcomes. Equally, academic public health needed an appreciation of service issues where research evidence would help. New generations of the public health workforce needed access to

---

[155] Personal communication, 2013.

good-quality teaching and education if they were to be well-prepared for challenging roles in the workplace.

The agendas across service and research appeared, however, to have widened, with academic departments focused on achieving high Research Assessment Exercise (RAE)[156] ratings linked to clinical epidemiology. The replacement of the research-based Part II examination at the FPH with observed practice led to less contact between public health trainees and academic departments of public health in some places. There were concerns about the quality of some Masters in Public Health degrees offered and also about the public health teaching content for medical and other health professional undergraduates. Although academic research fellowships started to be offered for public health trainees, this only applied to those from a medical background. The early PCTs were mostly too small to provide sufficient scale for public health research projects. Some of these issues were later picked up in the consultation document on the public health workforce in 2012 (DH, 2012b).

A halt to the steady progress

Between 2000 and 2008, there had been steady progress in multidisciplinary public health development at specialist level, and the beginnings of development for practitioners and the wider workforce in a period marked by substantial agreement across national public health organisations – including the FPH, UKPHA, Chartered Institute of Environmental Health (CIEH), the Royal Institute of Public Health (RIPH) and the Royal Society for the Promotion of Health (RSPH) – all working with the DH (largely representing the views of the four UK Health Departments) over what was needed. Even the BMA had recognised, if not welcomed, the presence of a multidisciplinary specialist workforce. There was also a willingness to work together. The FPH, for example, devoted its newsletter to members (*Ph.com*) in June 2006 to changes affecting the whole of the public health workforce, with sections on specific areas of practice and UK countries. By then, the FPH had over 3,000 members, one third of whom were from backgrounds other than medicine, and had closed its Specialist Development Committee. It was deemed no longer necessary as full integration of specialists had already taken place. Gradually, the need for having two FPH assessors on appointments panels for consultants

---

[156] High ratings are linked to better opportunities for further research grants. The. RAE is now known as the Research Excellence Framework (REF).

and DsPH (one statutorily required for medical appointments; the FPH opting to have a second advising on appointments of specialists) was dropped in favour of one, again because the second was no longer deemed necessary.

From 2008, the climate for development changed and there was a gradual lessening of availability of central DH funding for public health development as cuts around the health system started to bite. This latter period was also marked by increased dissonance across the national public health organisations. Hunter et al (2007) comment on the start of fragmentation of different voices claiming to speak for public health – the FPH, RIPH, RSPH,[157] UKPHA and CIEH.

The following year, matters became worse, with the demise of the UKPHA, which ceased to be an independent body in 2011 as a result of the cessation of DH funding, with some functions being absorbed into the FPH. As a result, following the March 2010 UKPHA conference, there was no longer a major national annual forum for multidisciplinary public health, with the FPH annual conference perceived by many to represent only those working at, or in formal training for, consultant/specialist practice.

By the beginning of the next decade, the fragmentation and lack of central investment in development increased further, when the publication of the incoming Coalition government's White Papers on health service and public health reforms in 2010 presaged the start of a two-and-a-half-year transition to new structures (DH, 2010a, 2010b).

A decade of change for specialists

The years 2000–2008 were marked by a substantial change for the public health workforce in the context of continuing health service reorganisations following the coming together of government policy aiming to tackle, for the first time, health inequalities, support across the four UK countries, DH funding for development and implementation of new initiatives, a willingness of national public health organisations to work together, and a groundswell of pressure for change from the service public health sector in particular.

Two FPH Presidents during this period commented on the length of time needed to deliver change. From their perspective, one presidential term of three years was insufficient – it needed a run of presidents sympathetic to the notion of a multidisciplinary public health workforce

---

[157] As part of a rationalisation exercise of June 2007, the RIPH and RSPH announced their intention to merge.

to enable change to become fully embedded.[158] Somervaille et al (2007) commented on the importance of having support from people in strategic positions within the DH in delivering these changes. They stated that all four UK Departments of Health were 'critical both financially and more importantly for the strategic policy statement it conveyed' (p 412). A former CMO also felt that the support from the RDsPH group should not be underestimated. The corporate group of RDsPH met monthly with the CMO: 'if I asked them to do something they would usually do it. Most were on the side of multidisciplinary public health but some went out of their way to find non-medical people'.[159] As another interviewee put it: 'for a long while, those of us medics who sincerely favoured a multidisciplinary workforce were in a small minority, despite growing lip service to the cause as it became politically correct to be seen to support this approach'.[160]

Key achievements

- Non-medical appointments at consultant level.
- A cadre of non-medical DsPH.
- A substantial increase in senior-level public health capacity and competency.
- Investment in building public health capacity and capability at the senior level.
- A shared view of what constituted public health practice.
- More prominence for senior public health roles.

Learning points

- A decade when there was the right climate for change.
- Perceived threats were still holding doctors back – constant reorganisation.
- Pressure from reorganisation to fill an increased number of senior public health posts.
- Substantial increase in the specialist public health workforce at a critical time in meeting increased demand for public health skills.
- The DH was on board with funding for development, nationally coordinated with local flexibility.
- Competencies/equivalence of standards were a key unifying force across the workforce.

---

[158] Personal communication, 2013; McEwen, Witness Seminar 2, in Evans and Knight (2006, p 82).
[159] Personal communication, 2012.
[160] Personal communication, 2012.

- Pay is an important issue for perceived equality for specialists – access, opportunity and achievement.
- There was no overall strategic framework for the whole of the public health workforce. The public health workforce plan was never published.
- There was no clear idea of how to retain cohesion across a dispersed public health workforce – networks were one answer, although there was no common agreement.[161]

---

[161] This issue arose again as part of the Coalition government's reforms (see Chapter Eight).

FIVE

Changes for specialists II: The new regulatory system for specialists

Introduction

For doctors, at the end of the 1990s, the standard, statutory process for achieving inclusion in the Specialist Register of the General Medical Council (GMC) and thereby becoming eligible to apply for NHS consultant posts was via satisfactory completion of specialist training in public health medicine. A similar process was introduced by the General Dental Council (GDC) for dentists becoming consultants in dental public health. This process was in line with the training requirements for all medical specialties, with each Royal College or Faculty setting its curriculum to be approved by the GMC. With recognition of public health specialists from backgrounds other than medicine it became clear that an equivalent regulatory system for assuring quality and protecting the public would be required for all those specialists who were not regulated by the GMC or the GDC.

This chapter:

- describes the identification of the need for professional regulation of the new cohort of non-medically or dentally qualified public health specialists;
- outlines the establishment of the new regulatory processes and registration for non-medical public health specialists;
- describes the creation and role of the UK Voluntary Register for Public Health Specialists (UKPHR); and
- explains the emergence of defined specialists among the multidisciplinary specialist workforce.

Setting up the regulatory processes

It was recognised within the Department of Health (DH) that the creation of Director of Public Health (DPH) posts that could be occupied, from 2002, by suitably competent individuals from a wide range of professional backgrounds carried with it new risks. These included the absence of professional accreditation or recognition for non-medically qualified specialists, and, in particular, the absence of any regulatory framework.

Until then, professional regulation under the jurisdiction of the DH had been restricted to health professionals who had contact with individual patients, whose actions could be interpreted as assault if conducted ineptly or inappropriately. Specialist public health practice was distinctly different as its proponents rarely had dealings with individual patients or clients and it took some time to gain consensus on the notion that a public health specialist's impaired fitness to practise could adversely affect the health or well-being of whole communities, rather than simply named individuals. When this consensus was reached, it was agreed that some form of regulation was required in order to protect the populations served by this new, so far completely unregulated, group of DsPH. There was, in addition, pressure from some medically qualified DsPH that their non-medically qualified peers should be regulated in an equivalent manner to their own professional regulation by the General Medical Council (GMC).

As a matter of policy, the DH required any new regulator to be established in voluntary form in order for the national criteria for regulation to be met, primarily to demonstrate that a new professional group was being established and that it would be sustainable and required professional regulation.

A team from the London School of Hygiene and Tropical Medicine, led by Klim McPherson, had been commissioned by the DH to undertake the feasibility study of the case for national standards of public health practice (Lessof et al, 1999). Their report provided clear evidence of the potential for multidisciplinary public health practice at consultant level. The conclusions of the feasibility study were accepted by the DH and provided a helpful basis on which to move forward.

After the publication of the feasibility study, the Tripartite Group was set up, involving the Faculty of Public Health (FPH), Multidisciplinary Public Health Forum (MDPHF) and Royal Institute of Public Health (RIPH), each of which had two representatives, as well as representation from the UK Health Departments. In addition, there was an Advisory Group chaired by the former Chief Medical Officer (CMO) Kenneth Calman. The intention was for the Tripartite Group to develop plans for an equitable and proper professional structure, including regulation, for specialists from backgrounds other than medicine. Following Lord Hunt's (2001) speech and the publication of 'Shifting the balance of power' (DH, 2001, 2002a), DsPH from backgrounds other than medicine began to be appointed and the requirement for regulation became a high priority.

The Tripartite Group's progress had been faltering and slow – tensions were high between the FPH, with its representation of a still largely medical membership, and the MDPHF, whose membership wanted to see rapid change and a confirmed professional identity. The RIPH, which had always had a broad, multidisciplinary membership, acted as an honest broker but with limited influence and no authority within the Tripartite Group. Only when the DH provided independent support to the work of the Tripartite Group and a clear deadline for completion of its deliberations, with the expectation of a plan to open a new register for public health specialists from backgrounds other than medicine, did it deliver, with the resulting recommendation to establish a voluntary register for specialists from backgrounds other than medicine and dentistry.

By 2002, getting resolution of the issues that would lead to full recognition and regulation of specialists in public health from backgrounds other than medicine had become a priority for the DH, in particular, because of the issue of public protection in the case of unregulated non-medical DsPH. This was supported by Don Nutbeam, who, as Head of Public Health, was the most senior member of the then CMO Liam Donaldson's public health team from a non-medical background. So, with independent facilitation and support to the Tripartite Group, after several months, its goals were achieved with full consensus.

The next step was to establish regulation as an independent entity. The FPH had wished to oversee regulation itself, but there were two main objections to this at the time: first, there was a lack of trust among the workforce that the FPH had the interests of multidisciplinary public health specialists at its heart; and, second, the idea of having a combined professional body and regulator was not supported centrally. Within the DH, then as now, there was a debate as to whether public health specialists presented a significant risk to the public and, thus, whether regulation was needed at all. But, eventually, it was agreed to proceed with the opening of a UK-wide voluntary register.

The UK Voluntary Register for Public Health Specialists (subsequently to become known as the UK Public Health Register [UKPHR]) was officially launched at the UK Public Health Association (UKPHA) conference in March 2003 by the then Minister for Public Health Hazel Blears. The announcement was greeted with delight by public health specialists and trainees[162] from backgrounds other than medicine as a first and important step in promoting equity of status between medically qualified and other public health specialists.

The first chair of the UKPHR was James (Jim) McEwen, a former President of the FPHM. Interestingly, despite being a doctor and former FPHM President, his appointment was widely welcomed by the multidisciplinary community as he was considered a person of professional integrity with a firm belief in the multidisciplinary nature of public health, as well as being respected by the FPHM rank and file.

The UKPHR was established as a limited company and with all of the infrastructure required of a regulator, including a board of management, trained, independent 'fitness to practise' panels, and independent, volunteer portfolio assessors. To date, it has not been necessary to invoke its full disciplinary powers, but they remain ready to be used if required.

The establishment of the UKPHR was a significant landmark for multidisciplinary public health – for the first time in the UK, all public health specialists could explicitly demonstrate adherence with national standards equivalent to the standards expected of medically qualified public health specialists. With full support of the MDPHF, the UKPHR established strict criteria for registration, and rejected the notion of a 'grandparenting clause'[163] for established specialists, requiring every applicant to complete its onerous portfolio assessment.[164] The framework for assessment needed to meet rigorous standards but, at the same time, be 'doable'. Assessors were appointed from among volunteer professional and lay people, trained to undertake assessment against the set criteria for registration.

By the end of 2003, at least six people had been accepted on the UKPHR through the portfolio route.[165] Aspiring non-medical specialists started to prepare early on in anticipation of the opening of the UKPHR. All non-medical DsPH, upon appointment, were offered provisional registration with the UKPHR, pending putting together a portfolio for assessment.

---

[162] The setting up of training schemes is covered in Chapter Six.

[163] A mechanism for automatic recognition of status.

[164] The framework for assessment was developed by a team led by the Public Health Resource Unit (PHRU) and based on the FPH 'Record of in-Training Assessment' competencies and Part I knowledge requirements. This framework was also used by the FPH for a number of years for portfolio assessment of overseas medics seeking public health registration in the UK.

[165] 'Minutes of the meeting of the Faculty of Public Health Executive Committee', 11 December 2003, FPH archives, Box Reference 375789133.

This retrospective portfolio assessment route was closed to all but exceptional cases in 2006, being largely superseded by what is known as the 'standard' route, comprising satisfactory completion of specialist training and having passed the full membership examinations of the FPH. The retrospective route, however, provided a serious boost to accredited senior capacity by 2007/08, when over 400 specialists had been registered with the UKPHR as 'generalists'.

All registrants were required, from the outset, to remain up to date with their continuing professional development. This was in line with requirements for doctors registered with the GMC or dentists with the General Dental Council (GDC). In addition, the UKPHR intends to introduce formal revalidation arrangements for public health specialists, again in alignment with requirements for public health doctors.[166]

Defined specialists

Soon after the opening of the UKPHR, it became clear that many well-established public health specialists would not be able to achieve completion of the retrospective portfolio assessment required for entry. On analysis, it was recognised that a cohort of highly specialised people from backgrounds other than medicine would fall outside the requirements for registration. After long, hard deliberation, the UKPHR board made the decision to establish a second type of specialist registration for 'defined specialists', which would be equivalent in status to generalist specialist registration but be for those whose specialisation had normally occurred earlier in their careers, and certainly well before any notion of access to specialist public health training existed, resulting in competent practice in a narrower and more specialised area of practice than that expected of 'generalist' specialists.

The UKPHR opened for registration of defined specialists in April 2006, with assessment being by retrospective portfolio assessment against a specifically provided framework, again developed by the Public Health Resource Unit (PHRU). At the time, this decision was made with the support of the then FPH Vice-President. The possibility of the development of a higher specialist training route for those seeking defined specialist registration was also being discussed, with the expectation that, as with generalists, the retrospective route would only be open for a limited period of time pending the opening of formal training routes (apart from exceptional cases). In the event,

---

[166] For a statement on UKPHR policy with regard to revalidation, see: www. publichealthregister.org.uk/node/220 (accessed April 2014)

this did not take place and the retrospective route has remained the only possibility for recognition at specialist level for those in defined areas of public health practice.

However, this decision was, and still is, contentious. Only in mid-2013 did the FPH decide to offer defined specialists membership of the FPH, while generalist specialist registrants are routinely offered fellowship. There are many people who remain uncomfortable at the equivalence given to defined specialists, given their lack of experience across the whole of public health practice: while they are required to demonstrate the same level and breadth of knowledge of public health as their generalist colleagues, they are not expected to be able to demonstrate practical experience (knows/shows how) of all the competency areas. They are, however, required to demonstrate a higher level of competency than a generalist in specific areas of practice.

To date, the number of defined specialists on the UKPHR is not large, 51 compared with 312 via the generalist specialist route as at September 2013.[167] Defined specialists are most numerous in the fields of health protection and health intelligence. A small number have been able to demonstrate the competencies required of a DPH and have thrived in such roles, while most continue in their chosen specialist field of work.

Academic public health remains a gap in specialist registration as there is little to commend registration to academic staff from non-medical backgrounds. Medical staff, even if working in a pure research setting, are likely to see the benefits of medical regulation, which, through provision of specialist advice to the National Health Service (NHS), allows them access to honorary NHS consultant status and, hence, to Clinical Excellence Awards, while no such benefits exist for non-medical academics. As the proportion of non-medical public health academics grows, there may be cause to revisit the benefits of NHS – or local authority – attachments, or otherwise risk losing much of the added value that academics bring to local public health practice.

The future of specialist regulation

Regulation provides protection for the public in that regulated professionals are required to meet specific standards and ethical practice and can be removed from registers if they are deemed not to meet required standards and behaviour. The future of specialist regulation in multidisciplinary public health is not, as yet, finalised.

---

[167] Personal communication with UKPHR chief executive officer, October 2013.

—

The usual pattern for professional regulation of health professionals has been for voluntary registration followed by consideration of statutory regulation only once sufficient numbers have been generated and there is a clear case for statutory regulation.

The UKPHR was established in 2002 and accepted registrants from May in that year. In 2010, the DH commissioned a review of regulation of public health professionals, which was conducted by Gabriel Scally (then Regional Director of Public Health for the South West). The review report (DH, 2010c) recommended statutory regulation by the Health Professions Council (recently renamed the Health and Care Professions Council [HCPC]) for non-medical 'generalist' specialists. It did not find the case proven for either defined specialists or public health practitioners. One early option considered by Scally for regulation of specialists from multidisciplinary public health backgrounds was with the GMC, but the GMC was not in favour of this.

It seems clear, however, that this is not yet the end of the story. The 'Parliamentary Health Committee twelfth report',[168] which considered the Coalition government's public health reforms, came out in favour, on the basis of the evidence it received, of statutory regulation with the HCPC but commented that the government was still sceptical, its preferred approach being to ensure effective and independently assured voluntary regulation. This was evident in the public health White Paper *Healthy lives, healthy people* (DH, 2010b), incidentally issued on the same day as the Scally Report (30 November 2010), which, in its consultation questions at the end of the document, asked for views on voluntary regulation.

The FPH's formal position has consistently been in favour of statutory regulation. The UKPHR, if voluntary regulation does not continue, would wish to become the statutory regulator of multidisciplinary public health specialists. The UKPHR has raised concerns about potential regulation by the HCPC: first, public health would be a very small discipline within the HCPC; second, the HCPC has no published plans to introduce revalidation;[169] and, third, the UKPHR is concerned

---

[168] Issued 19 October 2011. Available at: www.publications.parliament.uk/pa/cm201012/cmselect/cmhealth/1048/104802.htm (accessed December 2013). Chapter Eight sets out in full the Coalition government's reforms and assesses the implications for public health.

[169] Revalidation is a requirement by the GMC for all practising registered doctors to ensure that they are safe to practise and up to date in their knowledge and skills.

that regulation of specialists by the HCPC would 'block a developing "skills ladder" between practitioners and consultant grade staff'.[170]

Much of the debate has centred round two points: first, the need for protection of the public and the risks of having a senior professional group in positions of influence who are statutorily unregulated in terms of standards and ethical practice; and, second, the issue of equity between qualified medical and non-medical professionals at the specialist level of practice. In order to practise, public health doctors are required to be regulated as specialists through the statutory mechanism of the GMC. It could be argued that it makes little sense to have non-medical public health specialists fulfilling identical roles in the workforce with a requirement only for voluntary regulation.

Confusion around this issue has come to the fore since the implementation of the Coalition government's reforms for public health and the transfer of substantial numbers of health service public health staff to local government employment. Whereas senior public health appointments in the health service since 2002 have included the requirement for voluntary regulation for non-medical specialists, to date, there is no such requirement imposed upon local authorities. There have been reported appointments to senior public health responsibilities in local government during 2013 where individuals have not been qualified to specialist status and therefore not subject to regulation.

A further issue associated with statutory regulation of health professionals is the notion of a protected title. This requires primary legislation. There is currently no protected title for a non-medical specialist in public health. While employed within the health service, senior public health staff reaching the senior levels (8d or 9[171]) could use the title of 'consultant' from the (Agenda for Change) profile for that level. Since April 2013, there are very few senior public health staff employed within the health service. It is unclear whether this issue is more easily resolved if the HCPC or the UKPHR were to be the statutory regulator.

In 2013, the Minister for Public Health announced that statutory regulation by the HCPC was the way forward. At the time of writing this chapter, a consultation is awaited from the DH on the precise arrangements for multidisciplinary specialist regulation in the future.

---

[170] Letter from the UKPHR chair to all registrants, January 2014. Personal archive of the authors.

[171] Agenda for Change bands span 1–9, with band 8 split into four (8a–d), that is, 12 levels in total.

Key achievements

- UK-wide Voluntary Register for Public Health Specialists established.
- Specialist regulation introduced in June 2003.
- Identification and registration of defined specialists followed generalists on the UKPHR.

Learning points

- Creation of a new group – defined specialists – within the profession triggered new anxieties.
- Employers willing to appoint medical and non-medical specialists.
- Portfolio assessment is complex and labour-intensive for both applicants and assessors.

SIX

Changes for specialists III: The establishment of multidisciplinary higher specialist training in public health

Introduction

A core component within the multidisciplinary public health agenda from the start was to widen training opportunities for public health practitioners outside medicine with an eye to breaking the glass ceiling in public health at the highest level. The early 1990s had seen the opening up of Master's courses in public health to those without a medical degree but the route to specialist jobs in public health was exclusively through specialist registration with the General Medical Council (GMC), which was normally achieved via a formal training scheme in public health medicine that was only open to medical graduates.

Following the publication of *Saving lives: our healthier nation* (DH, 1999a), as we have seen earlier, public health consultant posts in health authorities began to be advertised to suitable candidates both with or without medical qualifications, and in 2003, a retrospective route to voluntary specialist registration via portfolio assessment was opened for senior non-medical people in public health, previously working, but not previously recognised as being, at specialist level. This was seen as a time-limited, 'catch-up' exercise, and those working to develop the public health workforce foresaw the need to develop, in parallel, a prospective training route to specialist appointments to develop the next generation of multidisciplinary public health specialists. It is the evolution of these multidisciplinary higher specialist training schemes that is the focus of this chapter.

As will be shown, the creation of a single, nationwide multidisciplinary higher specialist training scheme in public health took a number of years. It evolved in a piecemeal fashion against the backdrop of the rising attention being paid to the inequalities in training, development and accreditation of those working in public health outside of medicine, and the work of the Multidisciplinary Public Health Forum (MDPHF) and the Tripartite Group outlined earlier in the book. Many of the early training schemes for those from backgrounds other than medicine that emerged little resembled their medical counterparts, but, over time, they evolved into something that was equivalent and, later, fully integrated with medical training in public health: a unique outcome within a medical specialty.

> **This section covers:**
>
> - the context of medical training in public health;
> - the early development of ad hoc training for non-medics in public health;
> - the gradual transition to a common approach for non-medical training; and
> - the move to a single public health training model for medics and non-medics.

Setting the context: medical training in public health

At the end of the 1990s, the standard route for doctors to be eligible to apply for consultant posts in public health was via satisfactory completion of specialist training in public health medicine and inclusion on the Specialist Register of the General Medical Council (GMC). This process was in line with the training requirements for all medical specialties. Doctors were eligible to apply to enter specialist training in public health medicine if they had completed a minimum of three years' full-time equivalent in approved medical training posts. These dedicated specialist training schemes were managed by the Postgraduate Deaneries, the national network of bodies responsible for overseeing postgraduate medical and dental education and training throughout the UK.

Public health training was (and remains) formally a four-year programme, to which most programmes added a fifth year near the beginning of training, in which trainees were expected to study for a Master's degree in public health (or, in some deaneries, a closely allied approved course, such as epidemiology; or, historically, Consortium training comprising content delivered by several providers). During their time on the training programme, trainees (known as registrars, as in all medical specialties at the time) would be required to pass the Faculty of Public Health Medicine (FPHM) examinations (then known as Parts I and II) and to be assessed as having made adequate progress and have signed off a suite of competencies relevant to public health practice. Typically, trainees processed through several attachments during their time on the training programme, to ensure breadth of experience. Such attachments could include time in approved placements in an

Table 6.1: The establishment of the first multidisciplinary public health training schemes in England and Wales

Region/deanery	Year of first scheme	Number of trainees (first cohort)	Length of first schemes
North West	1999 pilot, established 2000	5	4 years
West Midlands	1999 pilot, established 2000	2	3 years
South West	1999	2	3 years
Trent	1999/2000	6	2 years
London	2000	4	4 years
Eastern/East of England	2001	2	3 years
Kent, Surrey & Sussex	2002	2	Unknown
East Midlands	By 2002	2	Unknown
Oxford	2002	1	5 years
Wessex	2003	4	5 years*
North East	2003	Unknown	5 years*
Yorkshire & Humber	Around 2003	Unknown	5 years*
Wales	2004	3	5 years

Note: *Where the length of the first scheme is unknown but it was set up around 2003, after the opening of Part II, it is assumed that it followed the model of other regional schemes and lasted five years.

Also note that Trent was later split between East Midlands and Yorkshire and Humber.

Sources: Table compiled from: Cornish and Knight (2002); Pilkington et al (2007); personal communications, 2011, 2013; Brown and Learmonth (2005); Reports of the Faculty of Public Health Medicine visits to North West region/Mersey Deanery 12–13 November 2001; West Midlands 12–13 September 2000 and 20–21 September 2001; Trent Deanery 21–22 October 1999; London/Kent, Surrey and Sussex 22–23 November 2001. FPH archives, Box Reference 375789159; 'Minutes of the meeting of the Trainee Members Committee', 10 June 2002; 'Papers of the Trainee Members Committee meeting', 2 December 2002. 'Minutes of the meeting of the Trainee Members Committee meeting', 4 March 2002. Box Reference 375789136.

academic department or overseas, for example. At the end of training, trainees were awarded their Certificate of Completion of Specialist Training (CCST). Registrars would be offered full membership of the FPHM upon passing the membership examinations – this was separate from, and often predated, completion of specialist training. Acquisition of the CCST was accompanied by recommendation of the individual by the FPHM for entry onto the GMC specialist register.

Eligibility to apply for consultant in public health posts in the NHS was dependent on holding a CCST or being certified as within three months of achieving this.

Dentists training in dental public health followed an equivalent higher specialist training route as public health doctors, leading to registration with the General Dental Council (GDC) and eligibility for both consultant in dental public health and consultant in public health medicine posts.

The development of early regional public health training schemes for those from backgrounds other than medicine

Following the publication in the mid- to late 1990s of local public health workforce surveys and training needs assessments, such as the one commissioned by the Regional Director of Public Health in the West Midlands discussed earlier (Somervaille and Griffiths, 1995), some regions began to explore ways to improve training and support for wider public health staff from backgrounds other than medicine. The North West and West Midlands, for example, piloted embryonic training schemes whereby a couple of individuals a year were funded, usually through the health authorities, to study for a Masters in Public Health while gaining some service experience (McErlain, 1998; Cornish and Knight, 2002). To further support similar bursary schemes, in 1998 the NHS Executive allocated a two year public health development fund to improve capacity and capability in public health, for which Regional Offices had to bid. In some regions these funds were used to set up training programmes for multidisciplinary public health trainees (McErlain, 1998; Cornish and Knight, 2002).

While these small-scale initiatives were taking shape, discussions began about creating a formal national or regionally coordinated specialist training programme for non-medics in public health. A report produced for the Regional Directors of Public Health (RDsPH) in 1998, for example, looking at the status of national and local initiatives for the development of public health professionals outside medicine, highlighted the need for a national initiative for non-medical public health development, including a properly funded specialist training programme for public health practitioners linked to a career pathway (McErlain, 1998).

By 1999, two further enablers were in place to facilitate the development of regional training schemes for future public health specialists from backgrounds other than medicine: the first open sitting of the Faculty of Public Health Medicine (FPHM) Part I examination took place in 1999[172] (following the FPHM Annual General Meeting vote in 1998), as did the announcement in *Saving lives: our healthier nation* (DH, 1999a) that there would be a new cadre of 'Specialists in Public Health' within the NHS, which would be equivalent to medically qualified Consultants in Public Health Medicine. As a result of these developments, public health professionals without a medical degree could now work towards a professional qualification in public health and the seeds were being sown for that qualification to be linked to a career pathway that was to be multidisciplinary to the highest level.

The pace at which the early multidisciplinary schemes developed across the regions varied (as shown in Table 6.1) and depended upon a combination of factors, including funding availability[173] and capacity within health authorities to support additional trainees. They were initially set up to last between two and four years and usually incorporated a Masters in Public Health and at least one service placement (Cornish and Knight, 2002). They were, in the main, completely separate from their medical counterparts: they were funded differently and mostly of shorter duration, and had separate recruitment processes, fewer training opportunities and different exit points. Until the FPHM voted to open its Part II membership examination, Part I was the usual exit point for most multidisciplinary training schemes, which it was expected to take trainees between two and three years to reach. Following the FPHM membership agreement to open Part II in 2001, most regions sought funding to extend their schemes to five years to allow candidates to prepare for and sit the examination (Cornish and Knight, 2002).[174]

As new exit points emerged, the existing schemes were extended: one of the first multidisciplinary trainees interviewed for this book commented: 'we were on initially for two years. Once we'd done Part I we knew almost immediately we were going to be able to do Part II ...

---

[172] 'Minutes of the Faculty of Public Health Medicine Education Committee', 20 January 1999, FPH archives, Box Reference 375789135.

[173] Funding came from the element of non-medical education and training funding annual allocations to regions over which they had discretionary spend and also directly from some health authorities which wanted to support the initiative to widen access to specialist training (eg in London).

[174] Reports of the Faculty of Public Health Medicine visits to London/Kent, Surrey and Sussex, 22–23 November 2001 and West Midlands, 20–21 September 2001, FPH archives, Box Reference 375789159.

it just kept opening'.[175] In time, all the schemes offered five years[176] of training, equivalent to the length of medical training programmes, but there remained variation between regions in the extent of integration with medical schemes.

Reducing inconsistency across the early schemes

Some deaneries integrated their training offer, if not from the start, then within the first couple of years of multidisciplinary training, combining seminars, training courses and placement opportunities, as well as methods of assessing competency (Cornish and Knight, 2002).[177] Some Training Programme Directors faced barriers from Directors of Public Health (DsPH) and/or academic institutions, who refused to take trainees who were not medically trained, although these were usually circumvented. One commented:'where a trainer felt unable to support a non-medical trainee we simply by-passed them'.[178] As people got used to these new cohorts of trainees and realised their competency, many of the barriers broke down,[179] and by 2002, many of the schemes were using the medical 'Record of in-Training Assessment' (RITA) competencies to assess their trainees on an annual basis, although some used revised versions for their multidisciplinary trainees (Cornish and Knight, 2002).

One of the more enduring challenges was setting up communicable disease control placements and, in particular, 'on-call' rotations for multidisciplinary trainees, which were a core part of medical training in public health (Cornish and Knight, 2002). This is possibly less surprising in that it was the most clinical aspect of training and was an area of opposition within wider debates around employing non-medical public health specialists. By 2002, it was reported within the FPHM that most regions were offering three-month communicable disease control placements but trainees had participated in on-call rotas in only a few regions due to a combination of shortages of suitable supervisors on local on-call rotas, views of individual Consultants in Communicable Disease Control (CCDCs), whether trainees had any type of clinical background and issues around indemnity (Cornish and

---

[175] Personal communication, 2011.

[176] Schemes were for four years but up to five years for candidates without a relevant equivalent qualification who needed to undertake a Masters in Public Health.

[177] Personal communication, 2011.

[178] Personal communication, 2011.

[179] Personal communication, 2011.

Knight, 2002).[180] Pay for out-of-hours on-call was similarly inconsistent, as one of the trainees interviewed for this study reflected: 'I did on-call at the beginning even though I didn't get paid because I didn't want to be seen as different; I didn't want to give anyone the excuse to say that my training wasn't up to scratch'.[181]

Following the creation of the Health Protection Agency (HPA) in 2003, the FPHM set up a Health Protection Working Party to look at training in health protection across its training schemes. Issues for specialist trainees remained slow to be resolved, however, and even as late as 2004, concerns were raised within the FPHM that of the four specialist trainees[182] due to complete their training that year, only one had been able to participate in on-call and have all their competencies signed off.[183] One trainee interviewed for this book reported having to wait until their final year of training to do their three-month stint in health protection.[184] In time, however, as with other issues, there was a gradual resolution, and health protection and on-call became core educational requirements for all trainees, whatever their background.

Even where training opportunities began to be integrated, establishing consistency in recruitment took longer, which was partly a reflection on how schemes were funded. One person at the Witness Seminar in 2005 remembered sitting in early interview panels where 'it was a case of, we've got this many posts, we've got this many applicants, we take the top ones and do it completely on merit'; in other places, they said: 'we're taking six doc[tor]s and we've got funding for two [non-medical] specialists and whatever the balance of skills they allocated in that way'.[185]

Unlike their medical peers, trainees from backgrounds other than medicine did not initially have national training numbers, a system which ensured that funding from the Department of Health (DH) went to local deaneries to support their training. Higher specialist training for public health doctors was funded through the Medical and Dental Education Levy (MADEL), which was separate from the Non-Medical Education and Training (NMET) fund, which existed

---

[180] 'Papers of the Trainee Members Committee meeting', 2 December 2002, FPH archive, Box Reference 375789136.

[181] Personal communication, 2011.

[182] 'Specialist trainees' was the name given to early multidisciplinary public health trainees; the medical trainees were known as 'specialist registrars', a name now adopted for all trainees in public health.

[183] 'Minutes of the Faculty of Public Health Medicine Education Committee', FPH archive, 7 July 2004. Personal communication with FPH, August 2011.

[184] Personal communication, 2011.

[185] Cornish, Witness Seminar 2, in Evans and Knight (2006, p 36).

for the wider workforce (and from 1998, could be used for training in public health) (McErlain, 1998; Cornish and Knight, 2002). Many of the early multidisciplinary schemes were funded using top-sliced NMET funds, supplemented by funding from the regional or local health authorities. Funding was not always recurrent and even where deaneries were successful at first in securing funding for training posts, issues sometimes emerged in terms of sustaining funding for subsequent cohorts of trainees (Cornish and Knight, 2002).[186]

The situation improved following the creation of Workforce Development Confederations (created to provide local leadership and direction for workforce planning and development), which were to be responsible for a newly combined Multi-Professional Education and Training Budget (MPET) from 2001 (DH, 2001). As a result of the merging of MADEL and NMET into a single MPET fund, it became easier for multidisciplinary training to be financed within the regions. This was furthered in 2003 with the announcement at the FPHM by the Lead Postgraduate Dean that there would be national training numbers (NTNs) for all trainees, including specialist trainees, and that more NTNs would be requested from the DH.[187]

Every medical specialty in England had a designated 'Lead Postgraduate Dean', who acted as an advocate to progress the specialty. The first Lead Dean for Public Health was Graham Winyard, a former Vice-President of the Faculty of Public Health (FPH) and former Deputy Chief Medical Officer for England, who embraced the need for widening access to specialist training, and his successor, Michael Bannon, continued that support, which was helpful in moving towards nationwide multidisciplinary recruitment. The Conference of Postgraduate Medical Deans of the United Kingdom (COPMeD), chaired at the time by Lis Paice (London), was also positively inclined towards this innovation in 'medical' training.

A further inconsistency within recruitment to the early schemes existed in their entry criteria: some schemes accepted recent graduates with limited work experience, whereas others expected trainees to have between two and five years of postgraduate experience in a field relevant to public health (Cornish and Knight, 2002).[188] The inadequate

---

[186] 'Papers of the Trainee Members Committee meeting', 2 December 2002, FPH archive, Box Reference 375789136.

[187] 'Minutes of the Faculty of Public Health Medicine Education Committee', FPH archive, 29 April 2003. Personal communication with FPH, August 2011.

[188] Reports of the Faculty of Public Health Medicine visits to London/Kent, Surrey and Sussex 22–23 November 2001 and North West/Mersey Deanery 12–13 November 2001, FPH archives, Box Reference 375789159.

assessment of academic capability in the recruitment to some of the early schemes meant that some trainees struggled with passing the FPHM examinations.[189] As such, the schemes became more prescriptive, and by 2002, most programmes required a good honours degree (passed at 2:1 or above) or an equivalent professional qualification, as well as four or five years of relevant, postgraduate work experience (Cornish and Knight, 2002).

Creating a national model for multidisciplinary training schemes

As multidisciplinary training schemes emerged, and expanded, there were calls from all sides for greater clarity and national consistency in the offer made to trainees. Training programme directors sought guidance from the FPHM on matters such as the competencies trainees should be assessed on, appropriate exit criteria for the schemes and whether communicable disease training and on-call experience were essential requirements.[190] These were matched by requests from trainees for training to be formalised in all regions, and for schemes to be equally funded with equivalent training opportunities[191] (Pilkington et al 2007).[192]

In response, several developments took place. There was a move to include the multidisciplinary public health specialist training posts within the standard FPHM quality assurance visits to specialist registrar (medical) training posts. Visitors assessing training posts had the ultimate sanction to recommend the withdrawal of training locations where there were serious problems. In the case of specialist trainees, it also provided the opportunity to compare and contrast the different schemes. Visits to specialist training posts were first piloted in the South West and North West in 2000. By the end of 2001, a specialist visitor was included in all routine FPHM visits (Cornish and Knight, 2002; FPHM, 2001).

---

[189] Personal communication, 2011.

[190] Personal communication, 2011.

[191] These were voiced initially through the Association of Public Health Specialist Trainees, a forum set up by specialist trainees to discuss training issues and provide mutual support, and latterly through the FPHM's Trainee Members Committee (which emerged in 2002 from the previous Specialist Registrar Members Committee to reflect the newly multidisciplinary membership).

[192] 'Minutes of the Trainee Members Committee', 4 March 2002, FPH archive, Box Reference 375789136; 'Minutes of the Faculty of Public Health Education Committee', 12 July 2001. Personal communication with FPH, August 2011.

In 2001, a Specialist Training Coordinating Group was set up at the FPHM to look into the emerging schemes. Parallel to this, the MDPHF and the FPHM's Honorary Members Committee commissioned a study to investigate how public health specialist trainees were being supported to proceed to Part II and identify any risks to the future funding of multidisciplinary training schemes (Cornish and Knight, 2002).[193] Both groups published reports in 2002, providing for the first time a clear overview of the status quo of the different schemes across the country and making recommendations for how they needed to move forward. These included recommending that schemes should: be advertised nationally with defined entry criteria; be recruited to using a rigorous selection process; be offered for five years, incorporating at least two training locations, as well as health protection experience; be assessed through the FPHM Parts I and II examinations and the RITA training competencies; culminate in the award of a Certificate of Completion of Specialist Training (CCST); and have secure central funding to allow equity of opportunity for trainees, covering, for example, salary, study requirements, travel expenses, on-call payments and overheads – in effect, that schemes were modelled on, and integrated with, medical training as far as possible.

As time went on, the differences between regional programmes became less marked. By 2005, there were schemes up and running in all regions in England and Wales (Griffiths et al, 2005). The specialist trainees proved themselves to be as competent as their medical counterparts in both the workplace and in examinations: the first non-medical trainees passed Part I in 2001 and then Part II in 2003 (Whittaker and Barnes, 2005; Pilkington et al, 2007). In 2005, the first specialist trainee to have completed higher specialist training and achieved a CCST was recommended by the FPHM for inclusion on the UK Voluntary Register for Public Health Specialists, as it was then known, which had become the new end point for training (launched in 2003). This was a remarkable achievement, a first within a formal specialist medical training programme, and was celebrated within the FPHM's quarterly newsletter (Somervaille, 2005).

The issue that, perhaps, took the longest to be fully resolved was the terms and conditions of specialist trainees, both in terms of equivalence with medical trainees and in having a uniform system across the country. This was not helped by a lack of consistent trade union representation

---

[193] 'Papers of the Trainee Members Committee meeting', 2 December 2002, FPH archive, Box Reference 375789136; 'Minutes of the Faculty of Public Health Education Committee', 12 July 2001 and 4 October 2001. Personal communication with FPH, August 2001.

for trainees or, indeed, for public health specialists from backgrounds other than medicine. Some had existing trade union membership from a previous role in health or elsewhere in the public sector, but many did not – unlike medical public health personnel, who were represented by the British Medical Association (BMA). From the schemes' early establishment there was a wide variety in the salaries of trainees, remuneration for out-of-hours on-call, allocation of travel expenses and study leave entitlements (Pilkington et al, 2007). It was not until April 2003 that a 'specialist trainee' job description and person specification was agreed nationally, which helped unify the expectations in the recruitment and training of specialist trainees.[194] Equivalence of salary took longer to achieve and was, in the end, determined as part of the wider project, outlined earlier in the book, to achieve equity in the salaries of public health specialists occupying consultant in public health roles in the NHS, enabled through the introduction of Agenda for Change in 2004 (Wright, 2007).

The impact of *Modernising medical careers* on integrating public health specialist training

While the aforementioned changes were taking place to establish a multidisciplinary higher specialist training pathway in public health, in reaction in the main to wider developments within multidisciplinary public health, changes were occurring to medical training in England that would impact upon public health training across the board and help forge greater integration between schemes in terms of both the curriculum and recruitment.

Following the establishment of the Postgraduate Medical Education and Training Board (PMETB)[195] in 2003 and the publication of *Modernising medical careers: the next steps* (DH, 2004a) a single, unifying framework for postgraduate medical education and training across the UK was developed. As well as amending the structure and length of training for doctors, PMETB required all Royal Colleges and Faculties to submit curricula defining the content of their training programmes. The FPH's new public health curriculum was put in place from August 2007 (the first year that the newly created Foundation 2 grade

---

[194] 'Minutes of the Faculty of Public Health Medicine Education Committee', FPH archive, 29 April 2003. Personal communication with FPH, August 2011.
[195] The PMETB has since merged with the GMC. See: http://www.gmc-uk.org/about/PMETB_archive.asp (accessed January 2011).

doctors[196] were able to apply for higher specialist training in public health). It was based on the original (medical) RITA competencies and was structured to lay out clearly what learning outcomes were needed at different stages of training. The new curriculum also reflected the national agreements reached in 2006 relating to competency across the whole of the public health workforce (further outlined in Chapter Seven), that is, replacing the former 10 key areas of public health with four core and five defined areas of practice. It represented the first combined curriculum outlining training requirements for all public health trainees: those from medical and other graduate backgrounds (FPH, 2006; Lock and Sim, 2009).

Around the same time, the FPH commissioned a review of their Part I examination, known as the Southgate Review. Alongside the requirements of PMETB, the findings of the Southgate Review provided an opportunity for the FPH to modernise its whole examination system (FPH, 2004, 2005, 2006). As a result, in 2005, the syllabus for Part I (the public health knowledge exam) was revised and renamed 'Part A'. The Part II examination, formerly comprising a dissertation and oral assessment, was redesigned as an Objective Structured Public Health Examination (OSPHE), known as 'Part B', testing candidates' ability to demonstrate 'show how' competency through a scenario-style examination based on real-life situations. It was envisaged that trainees would sit this second exam in their second or third year of training to allow a longer period post-FPH membership for trainees to develop the high-level skills needed to prepare them for their role as consultants.

Another consequence of *Modernising medical careers* (DH, 2004a) was the establishment of a national recruitment process in public health, aligned with all medical specialties, from application through to selection. Prior to national recruitment, most deaneries had their own recruitment processes, although there were some examples of joint-working. In the first years of national recruitment in public health (from 2008), deaneries formed recruitment clusters, which each used nationally consistent recruitment methods. Since 2011, this has moved

---

[196] *Modernising medical careers* (DH, 2004a) reformed the Senior House Officer medical grade, orienting training around competencies met rather than time-served in training, and reduced the total time spent in training before doctors became eligible for consultant posts. Following the changes, doctors entered a two-year foundation programme after graduation before selecting a career path through higher specialist training. The first foundation year was similar to what had been the Pre-registration House Officer year, after which doctors became registered with the GMC (Cooper, 2005).

to a single selection centre model, which is used for recruitment to all deaneries.[197] Significantly, the national method of selection that recruits candidates based on scores both at an assessment centre (incorporating numerical and verbal reasoning, and since 2011, situational judgement tests) and a selection centre (with an OSPHE–style multiple interview arrangement) has helped ensure consistency in recruitment across deaneries and greater equality between the selection of graduates from medical and other backgrounds. Since the introduction of central recruitment, deaneries have no longer been in direct control of their own recruits. For public health training, all shortlisted applicants are selected purely on interview and assessment performance, irrespective of professional background.

The changing profile of trainees over time

The first multidisciplinary schemes established from 1999 recruited between one and five candidates, but, due largely to funding uncertainties, not all schemes were able to recruit on an annual basis following their first cohorts of trainees. As might be expected, therefore, the body of trainees from backgrounds other than medicine took time to build up. By the time of the FPH's 2003 workforce report, there were 60 specialist trainees compared with 297 medical trainees training in public health in England (ranging from one to 17 per region).[198]

Figure 6.1 shows the new recruits to public health training between 2000 and 2013, using data from two different sources: the FPHM's (2005) workforce census (Gray and Sandberg, 2006) and recruitment data from the East Midlands Healthcare Workforce Deanery since national recruitment began in 2008.[199] The graph is striking in showing the gradual rise in the proportion of trainees recruited from backgrounds other than medicine from fewer than 14% in 2000 to 64% in 2011, although the proportion fell slightly in 2012 (61%) and again in 2013 (47%). Although 2013 was the first year to include Scotland, the number of trainees appointed to the scheme in Scotland was insufficient to be the reason for the shift downwards in the proportion of non–medics. Unfortunately, recruitment data was not available in this format for the years between 2005 and 2007. Without data for these intervening years, it is not possible to know in which year the

---

[197] Personal communication, 2011.

[198] Gray, S. and Perlman, F. (2004) 'Draft report on the public health workforce in the UK', in Papers for the meeting of the Faculty of Public Health Executive Committee, 27 January, FPH archive, Box Reference 375789133.

[199] Personal communication, 2013.

Figure 6.1: Public health recruitment between 2000 and 2004 and since national recruitment started in 2008, showing the breakdown between medical and other graduates

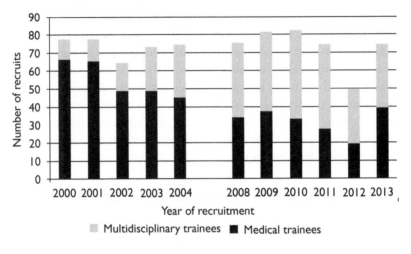

Note: The data from the workforce census (2000–04) includes data from England, Wales, Scotland and Northern Ireland (but only England and Wales were multidisciplinary, Wales from 2004); the data from national recruitment contains data from England and Wales only from 2008 to 2012, and then Scotland also in 2013.

ratio of new recruits switched for the first time in favour of those from backgrounds other than medicine, and whether the shift occurred following the move to national recruitment.

The majority of new training recruits over the last few years have been from backgrounds other than medicine. Although national data are not available on the total number of individuals currently in training from different backgrounds, it is likely that the majority will be from backgrounds other than medicine. Correspondence with current training programme directors confirmed that in some deaneries, the majority of trainees are non-medics and have been for a few years (although there is variation across deaneries),[200] and although only reflecting the trainees who responded, data from the FPH's workforce census suggested that even as early as 2007, the proportion of non-medical trainees may have been as high as 52% (Gray and Sandberg, 2008). If, as anticipated, results in examinations and in-training assessments, as well as drop-out rates, are similar across trainees of

---

[200] Personal communication, 2011.

different backgrounds, these findings are likely to have an effect on the future profile of qualified public health consultants in the workforce.

Historically, many doctors made the decision to enter public health after several years of post-qualification experience, something reflected in a cohort study of medical students published in 2011 (Goldacre et al, 2011). Since the changes brought about by *Modernising medical careers* (DH, 2004a), medical trainees select their future specialty at an earlier stage within their training than previously (at Foundation 2). Many doctors apply for training posts in a variety of specialties to ensure they remain employed as a doctor and if, for example, GP recruitment is finalised before public health recruitment, doctors may accept the offer that is in their hand rather than wait for the results of public health recruitment. There is also less flexibility recognised within medical training to move across specialties, and receive retrospective recognition for prior training. As a consequence, a concern has been raised that the likelihood of doctors applying for public health more heavily depends upon their exposure to public health at undergraduate and Foundation 1 levels, which have tended to be regarded as weak. Furthermore, although Foundation 2 applicants vary in their experience, and some doctors trained in other specialties do still apply for public health, many medical applicants are now more junior than previously and have had less clinical exposure, something that may affect the knowledge and experience they bring to the profession (Goldacre et al, 2011).[201]

As a result of the move of public health functions largely out of the NHS following the passing of the Health and Social Care Act 2012, another concern raised around medical recruits to public health training has been that fewer doctors might apply to train in public health (Packham and Robinson, 2011). This has not been borne out in practice, with the number of medical applicants not varying significantly in absolute terms. Since 2009, there have been significantly more applicants to public health higher specialist training from backgrounds other than medicine compared with medical applicants. Although fewer in number, however, over the last couple of years, a higher proportion of eligible medical applicants (those meeting the person specification) have been offered places compared with eligible non-medical applicants.[202]

The number of applicants applying to train in public health overall varies by year. At times of health service reorganisation, the numbers of applicants, particularly from non-medical backgrounds, has tended

---

[201] Personal communication, 2011.
[202] Personal communication, 2013.

to increase, with applicants attracted by the prospect of job security for at least five years.[203] The change from hard-copy applications to a web-based format has also meant that around a sixth of those applying to train are not eligible: potential applicants are more aware of the availability of jobs and put in a single application, with relative ease, for any training scheme in the country. There remains considerable variation in competition ratios between programmes and sub-programmes within deaneries.[204]

Data provided by the UK Public Health Register (UKPHR)[205] show that the number of specialist registrants at September 2013 stand at 511: 312 of whom came through the 'generalist' portfolio route to registration; 51 through the more recent 'defined' portfolio route; and 144 through higher specialist training schemes, known as the 'standard route'.[206] For the last few years, the standard route has been the main route to generalist registration, with the retrospective 'generalist specialist' portfolio route only available by exception. Although, to date, it is the portfolio route that has helped to bolster the number of multidisciplinary specialists working as consultants in public health (CPH) in the workforce, in the future, it will increasingly be the training scheme that defines the profile of the people in these roles. Figure 6.2 sets out the recruitment and training as it operates in 2014.

Reflections

The development of multidisciplinary higher specialist training in public health, whereby suitably qualified graduates from a wide range of backgrounds are eligible to train alongside doctors within a medical specialist training programme, is a unique achievement and one that, as this chapter has shown, took time and commitment to achieve. In the UK, we have gone from the position of having no specialist training opportunities for graduates from backgrounds other than medicine in 1998 to a position in 2013 where non-medical trainees have dominated recruitment numbers in recent years and make up the majority of those in training overall. Three of the four UK countries have opened their training schemes to non-medics, the exception being Northern Ireland (Scotland joined the multidisciplinary, national recruitment process for the first time in 2013), and since 2007, the route to specialist training

---

[203] Personal communication, 2013.

[204] See: http://www.fph.org.uk/applications_in_england%2c_scotland_and_wales (accessed March 2014).

[205] Personal communication with UKPHR chief executive officer, October 2013.

[206] There are also four members with dual registration.

Figure 6.2: Overview of the integrated higher specialist training programme for public health, 2014, from application to graduation

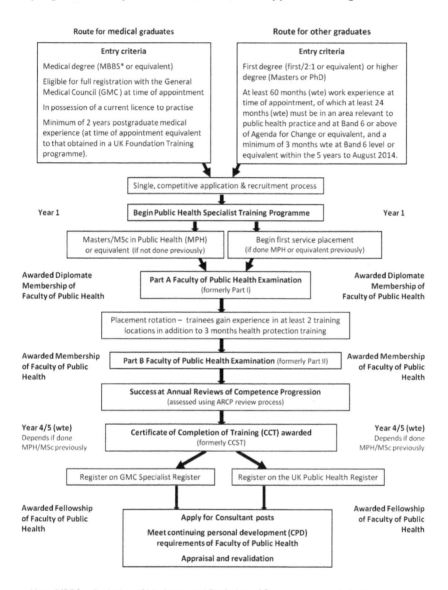

Note: MBBS – Bachelor of Medicine and Bachelor of Surgery; wte – whole-time equivalent.

Source: Diagram based on the 2014 National Personal Specification ST1 Public Health. Available at: www.fph.org.uk/applications_in_england%2c_scotland_and_wales (accessed March 2014) and the 2010 Public Health Training Curriculum. Available at http://www.fph.org.uk/training_downloads (accessed April 2014)

within the Defence Medical Services has been open to non-medical serving officers within the armed forces.[207] In due course, this will have a strong impact on the composition of public health specialists in the workplace.

Equivalent training schemes for those from backgrounds other than medicine did not emerge as a neat and uniform package, but evolved and expanded over time as new opportunities arose, such as the opening of the FPH examinations and the creation of the UKPHR. As a result of this piecemeal development, it is difficult to pinpoint the year in which it could be said that a national multidisciplinary public health training scheme emerged. By 2005, every English and Welsh region had a training scheme open to multidisciplinary trainees, which represents one key milestone. Another was the unification of the FPH's curriculum in 2007, which was shortly followed by the start of a national recruitment process in 2008. Recruitment, however, only became truly integrated with the development of a single assessment centre in 2011.

Much of the work that took place to develop higher specialist training for those outside medicine was about ensuring equivalence of opportunities. It could be questioned, however, whether there has been too much focus on gaining equivalence within a medical training model, which has perhaps placed restrictions on the schemes to always fully reflect the demands and opportunities within the public health workforce in practice.

The early training schemes were criticised for being too NHS- and medically focused (Evans and Dowling, 2002); some have even criticised the schemes for producing 'genetically modified doctors' and as not having made the most of the diverse backgrounds of trainees (Hunter et al, 2007). On the one hand, these criticisms have some truth. Trainees from other backgrounds were brought into a medical training model, which was overseen by a medical faculty. Many of the changes in the mid-2000s to the curriculum, examinations and even recruitment in public health were to meet the requirements outlined by the medical training board (PMETB). On the other hand, training has evolved to take account of wider developments in public health practice, many of which reflected the multidisciplinary public health agenda. These include, for example, the strengthening of competency requirements in management, leadership and partnership-working, and the division of public health competencies into 'core' and 'defined' groupings, developed as part of the registration process for the UKPHR and

---

[207] Personal communication, 2013.

subsequently incorporated into the training curriculum for all public health trainees.[208]

To ensure that doctors continued to be part of the public health workforce and that a two-tiered training structure did not emerge, it is difficult to see what alternative there might have been for public health training outside the existing medical model. Historically, the organisation of professional training for public health doctors has been closely modelled on the arrangements established for other clinical disciplines, and the structure of medical public health practice has been aligned with that in clinical disciplines involving similar procedures for making career appointments and similar pay scales. For most medically qualified public health workers, these arrangements have been seen as vital for the establishment of their professional integrity, and to continue to recruit doctors in public health, therefore, concessions inevitably have had to be made within the institutional structure of education and practice in public health.

As a result of using a medical training model, however, there remain issues for multidisciplinary trainees in training. For example, since September 2005, the PMETB (now absorbed within the GMC) has had responsibility for training visits, and, as such, quality assurance of non-medical specialist posts is only conducted on an informal basis (FPH, 2006).[209] Whereas the general public health training scheme is overseen by the FPH, a faculty of the Royal College of Physicians, two of the alternative training routes to public health specialist roles remain only open to those with a medical/dental background. Specialist training in dental public health is overseen by the Royal College of Surgeons and only open to qualified dentists who are registered with the General Dental Council. Academic Clinical Fellowship (ACF) posts are funded solely for doctors across a range of specialties, including public health, by the National Institute for Health Research (NIHR) and allocated to deaneries, which then appoint candidates in collaboration with universities. Seventy-five per cent of ACF training is spent in academic placements, with the remaining time spent in service placements.[210]

That being said, there have been benefits for the workforce in taking this route to professional training and accreditation: using the existing, rigorous and well-respected medical model of training, and putting multidisciplinary trainees through the same training and assessment process, has ensured that all graduates from the training

---

[208] Personal communication, 2011.

[209] Personal communication, 2011.

[210] Both these training routes qualify specialists to apply for consultant in public health roles.

scheme, irrespective of background, meet the core set of skills and competencies recognised as necessary to undertake public health specialist roles. As a result of this, public health now benefits from having trainees from a diverse range of backgrounds, including medicine, nursing, environmental and social sciences, epidemiology, and informatics, to name a few, who bring diverse perspectives, interests and skills over and above their assessed core levels of competency to their practice.

Hopefully, the history of the emergence and development of multidisciplinary training in public health does not end here. The training structure and curriculum for specialists in public health has evolved to reflect changes in public health practice, and continues to do so: in 2010, the curriculum was further updated, with more focus around leadership, management and interagency working to better reflect challenges faced by public health consultants in the workplace (Cole et al, 2011).[211] Further changes have since been needed to reflect the changing locations of public health service delivery now that Primary Care Trusts have been disbanded and the HPA has moved into Public Health England, a new national specialist agency for public health.[212]

Medical specialist training, which has historically provided the structure for all public health training, also continues to change. On 1 April 2013, the work of the deaneries was passed to 13 Local Education and Training Boards (LETBs) set up under the aegis of Health Education England (HEE). As a Special Health Authority, HEE provides national leadership for planning and developing the whole health care and public health workforce, regardless of the background and final career aspirations of staff. LETBs have a wider remit than deaneries, and oversee training for all health care staff to national standards, with an emphasis on multidisciplinary training – in which public health has led the way. There are further proposals for medical training in the 2013 Shape of Training review (Greenaway, 2013), which recognises the need for flexibility of training for junior doctors, which may make it easier for doctors to change specialties rather than being forced to abandon clinical work at such an early stage in their career.

As roles and interfaces within the new public health, NHS, local authority and health care workforce education structures in England continue to emerge, it remains to be seen how and in what direction

---

[211] Public health competency is likely to be further updated following the *Public health workforce strategy* for England published in 2013 (DH et al, 2013) (see Chapter Eight).

[212] For more detail on the updated public health system in England, see Chapter Eight.

the schemes will need to evolve. The FPH specialist public health standards apply to the workforce across the four UK countries. The difficulty in the future will be in ensuring competency, backed by training, which is flexible and robust enough to cope with the now very different and still evolving public health systems that specialists will need to work within across the UK countries.

Key facilitators in achieving equality in multidisciplinary and medical higher specialist training in public health:

- opening of Masters in Public Health courses (from 1990);
- opening of Part I (1999) and Part II (2002) FPHM examinations (now Part A and Part B);
- opening membership of the FPHM;
- membership and chairmanship of the FPHM's Trainee Members Committee (formally Specialist Registrar Members Committee) (2002);
- clarity and consistency of funding – national training numbers for all trainees from 2003;
- equality in job opportunities on qualifying – the opening of consultant and director of public health posts to those from backgrounds other than medicine;
- defined competencies and assessment methods for all specialists and higher specialist trainees (National Standards for Public Health);
- a means of registration (equivalent to the GMC for doctors) – UKPHR;
- equivalence in salary (Agenda for Change);
- first unified curriculum in public health – introduced in 2007, following PMETB;
- national recruitment process – from 2008; and
- single, national assessment centre – from 2011.

SEVEN

The focus on practitioners and the wider workforce

Introduction

The focus of the early 2000s was on developing the specialist role in public health for those from backgrounds other than medicine and ensuring that this was embedded in appointments and training and development processes, providing equivalence with public health doctors. From 2004, attention shifted to development of the rest of the public health workforce – practitioners delivering public health programmes on the ground (eg health promotion and health visiting staff) and the front-line so-called 'wider workforce', who could have an impact on the population's health through their roles (eg teachers, social care and health service staff) (Donaldson, 2001).

This chapter outlines:

- the context for addressing the development and competency needs of practitioners and the wider workforce;
- the start of voluntary regulation for the senior public health non-medical workforce working in defined areas of practice and the unregulated practitioner workforce; and
- the development of, and the prominence given to, the role of those in the wider public health workforce.

Rise of interest in developing and recognising specific public health practitioner disciplines and functions

Practitioners have been a much more complex group to both understand and support strategically, being diverse in function and in employing organisations, and being numerically much greater than specialists. Whereas some practitioners would remain, along with public health specialists, in Primary Care Trusts (PCTs) following the 2002 health service reforms (DH, 2002a), many were located in provider health organisations, local authorities, primary care and the voluntary and independent sectors.

The spur for the public health skills and knowledge development of practitioners and the wider workforce was, as with specialists, in response to government policy, this time the White Paper *Choosing health: making healthier choices easier* (DH, 2004b). There had been earlier recognition, in the Treasury reports of 2002 and 2004 (Wanless, 2002, 2004), that addressing only the development needs of specialists would not deliver the wholesale changes to population health which would ensure that the health service could be affordable in the future: the so-called 'fully engaged scenario' whereby the whole population took more responsibility for health and prevention and adopted healthier lifestyles. The 2004 White Paper was in response to this challenge and addressed the development of practitioners and the wider workforce.

There was fertile ground for these messages to fall upon, and a growing identity among different occupational groups of their allegiance to a public health workforce 'family'. As early as 1994/95, the survey conducted by Somervaille and Griffiths (1995) had identified over 1,000 people working in public health across the UK who were not within the public health medicine framework. Their follow-up survey in 1998 (Somervaille and Griffiths, 1998) began to group people more closely according to whether they were working on the service side, in health protection, health intelligence or health promotion, or whether they were working in academic public health.

The importance of the contribution of the public health workforce beyond public health consultants was subsequently confirmed in the Chief Medical Officer's (CMO's) project to strengthen the public health function in England (Donaldson, 2001). This categorised the workforce into three groups, comprising specialists and consultants at the strategic level, practitioners at the operational level, and the wider workforce, who can influence the health of the public through their roles, for example, as teachers and social workers, but who would not call themselves part of the public health workforce.

The public health skills audit (Burke et al, 2001), undertaken as part of the implementation of the 1999 White Paper *Saving lives: our healthier nation* (DH, 1999a), specifically included a number of key occupational groups as part of the public health workforce: nurses (health visitors and school nurses), health promotion specialists, environmental health officers, epidemiologists and public health information officers.

In developing the very detailed *National Occupational Standards for Public Health* (Skills for Health, 2004), Healthwork UK[213] worked

---

[213] Later to become Skills for Health, the sector skills council dealing with the health service.

with those in the field from diverse backgrounds to understand what competency was required to deliver a range of public health functions. One former Director of Public Health (DPH)[214] recalls being asked to undertake a public health skills audit for this project, whereby everyone in the health authority public health department had to maintain a diary logging their public health activities, including those working in health promotion, pharmacy, oral health, health intelligence and community development. The importance of having occupational standards for public health practice should not be underestimated. It provided the first competency framework for the practitioner public health workforce, spanning the 10 key areas of public health,[215] and was pitched at graduate level. It showed practitioners what competency was required across the 10 key areas of public health, and informed the content of relevant university and further education college courses.

However, the only formal recognition of practitioner status remained through the Chartered Institute of Environmental Health (CIEH) for environmental health officers and through the Nursing Midwifery Council (NMC) for public health nurses. Public health nutrition staff were voluntarily regulated by the Public Health Nutrition Society. All other public health practitioners, including health promotion and health intelligence staff, were unregulated, with no clear career or qualification routes, although many would have master's degrees relevant to public health.

The rise of the concept of specialists in defined areas of practice[216] and its impact on practitioners

Specialist practice, as defined by the Faculty of Public Health (FPH) and adopted by the UK Public Health Register (UKPHR), required competency across all the agreed 10 areas of public health practice. Most practitioners, however, worked in specific areas of practice, such as health intelligence, health protection, health improvement, research (academic public health) or health services. Debates began in the 2000s about whether and how competency in specific areas of practice should be recognised and developed. Further work was undertaken to capture and define specific workforce groups, some of whose members wished to ally themselves to public health.

---

[214] Personal communication, 2013.

[215] See Chapter Four.

[216] For the full history of registration of specialists in defined areas of practice, see Chapter Five on regulation.

Following the opening in 2003 of the UKPHR for registration of 'generalist' specialists, that is, those competent across all 10 key areas of public health at an equivalent level with public health doctors, the clamour started for recognition at a senior level equivalent to consultant status of those with expertise in specific areas of public health practice. According to Jones and Earle (2009), early critics of the UKPHR 2003 competency-based framework were concerned that all public health specialists were expected to be competent across all 10 key areas of public health. They argued that if a truly multidisciplinary approach were to be adopted, the competencies should be measured across a whole multidisciplinary public health team and not based purely on individuals.

From a very early stage, the UKPHR was interested in the concept of recognition at consultant level for specialists in specific (defined) areas of practice (McEwen, 2004). Griffiths and Sugarman's (2004) *Scoping study*, commissioned by the UKPHR and followed by the Public Health Resource Unit's (PHRU's) work to establish a competency framework for retrospective portfolio assessment of defined specialists, identified and confirmed a wide range of disciplines wishing to formally ally themselves with public health at specialist level. These included health psychology, health economics, public health management and public health nutrition, and went beyond groups already identified (health promotion, health intelligence, public health nursing, health protection and environmental health).

This work led to a need to redefine the 10 key areas of public health. In developing a framework for assessment that would meet competency needs for a very wide range of specific public health disciplines (up to 20), the PHRU quickly discovered that having health promotion and health protection within the same key area would not work. A national workshop in March 2006,[217] at which all the main national public health organisations, as well as the Department of Health (DH), were present, recognised that there were competencies common to all public health professionals, whatever field of public health they worked in, and competencies relating to specific areas of practice. This was an important advance in enabling a wide range of practitioners, as well as those in the 'wider workforce', to identify themselves more clearly with the public health function. These revised competencies were subsequently used by the UKPHR within its assessment framework

---

[217] Personal archive of the authors.

for defined specialists, and also informed the revised curriculum for the FPH higher specialist training scheme.[218]

The core and defined areas of public health practice (2006)[219]

Core areas (applying to anyone working in a public health field at whatever level):

- surveillance and assessment;
- assessing the evidence;
- policy and strategy; and
- leadership and collaborative working.

Defined areas (applying to those working in specific areas of practice at whatever level):

- health improvement;
- health protection;
- public health intelligence;
- academic public health; and
- health and social care quality.

Practitioner expectations for development and progression were still frustrated. The identification and opening up of specialist career channels to those from backgrounds from medicine had served to raise expectations of, and aspirations for, opportunities for their own progression among practitioners. The 'window' for retrospective assessment by the UKPHR by portfolio for 'generalist' specialists ended (apart from exceptional cases) in 2006, effectively closing that route to most senior practitioners. The requirements for defined specialist registration from 2006 were challenging, requiring 'super-specialist' knowledge and skills in defined areas of practice. In the event, by 2013, relatively few practitioners have achieved this level of registration compared with generalist specialists[220] and it is unknown how many are preparing portfolios. The standard/default route for

---

[218] The UKPHR has continued to retain the 10 key areas for its 'generalist' specialist retrospective portfolio assessment framework.

[219] Adopted by the FPH in its post-August 2007 curriculum, and forming the basis for development of the UK public health competency framework (see Skills for Health, 2008).

[220] At September 2013, 51 registered as defined specialists compared with 312 via the generalist specialist route (personal communication with UKPHR chief executive officer [CEO], October 2013).

formal development and recognition at specialist level (as a generalist specialist, ie, competent across all core and defined areas of practice) has remained the higher specialist training scheme, to which entry is highly competitive and restricted to around 70 new trainees in any one year.

The PCT and Strategic Health Authority (SHA) mergers, resulting from the 2006 health service reforms (DH, 2005), served to create, within larger public health teams, more assistant and deputy DsPH posts from backgrounds other than medicine, many of whom could not formerly have progressed to this level of seniority. There was a thirst among this group below specialist and consultant level for development, recognition and a proper career structure beyond the handful of practitioners who, from 2003, could reach specialist-level practice. There were still no formal development routes for recognition of the much larger practitioner workforce and, other than the scarce places on deaneries' specialist training schemes, little opportunity for career progression from practitioner to specialist despite obvious interest in the field.

Focus on specific initiatives for the development of practitioners following the 2004 White Paper

The situation changed for the better in 2005 following the publication of the White Paper *Choosing health* in 2004 (DH, 2004b), when the DH was able to use the opportunity for developing a population approach to healthy lifestyle behaviours, outlined in the White Paper, to peg and fund a number of different initiatives for the development of the whole of the public health workforce – the 'golden years', according to a former public health workforce lead.[221] From 2005, the DH funded a suite of major developments, which had a subsequent impact on different groups in the practitioner workforce. These developments included support for the health promotion workforce, developing a new health trainer workforce, developing a competency framework that would apply to different career levels in the workforce and supporting public health career and leadership development, the latter building on the programmes already taking place in London and the West Midlands. These years were also marked by continuing agreement across national public health organisations and a willingness to work together on shared development.

---

[221] Personal communication, 2013.

Health promotion

The first public health practitioner group to receive attention following the 2004 White Paper were health promotion specialists. The report *Shaping the future of public health: promoting health in the NHS* (Griffiths and Dark, 2005), the result of a two-year project, was issued by the DH in July 2005. This followed earlier scoping work in 2003 by Griffiths, in preparation for setting up the UKPHR, when she had found a demoralised health promotion workforce for whom the 'glory days' of the mid-1980s' programme Health for All by the Year 2000[222] (WHO, 1981) were long gone. Many dedicated health authority health promotion teams had been broken up in 2002 as a result of the health service reforms to create smaller PCTs, and a number of staff had moved into provider trusts. Griffiths and Dark's survey, which fed into the 2005 report, identified a specialised health promotion workforce in England and Wales of around 2,000 whole time equivalents contributing to health improvement. The report compared this numerically with the FPH's membership workforce report for 2004 of 600 NHS consultants and specialists (including DsPH) and 350–400 specialist registrar trainees (only a small number of whom would be working at any one time on health improvement programmes). On the basis of the 2005 report, the DH funded an annual conference for health promotion specialists to be able to meet to debate issues and to share good practice.

A new look at public health competencies

The next stage was to develop, across the newly specified core and defined areas of public health practice, public health competencies that addressed the needs of different practitioner levels in the workforce. In 2006, commissioned by the DH and working with the PHRU, Skills for Health commenced work on a competency framework that spanned the four core and five defined areas of practice competencies across nine 'career' levels, from direct entry to the workforce, to senior strategic roles, such as DPH. It also looked, for the first time, at competency requirements across the 'wider' workforce. This was different from their *National Occupational Standards for Public Health* (Skills for Health, 2004), which were much more detailed, related to the former 10 key areas of public health and based around a single point of graduate-level practice.

---

[222] The Health for All by the Year 2000 initiative, launched in 1981 by the World Health Organization (WHO), had as its programming goal to promote health and human dignity and enhance the quality of life

The resulting 'UK public health skills and career framework' (UKPHSCF) (Skills for Health, 2008) was published by Skills for Health in April 2008. This provided, for the first time, a comprehensive framework for practitioners (and, indeed, those in the wider workforce) to self-assess their level of competency against what was required at the level in the workforce within which they were operating. They had a much clearer idea of personal development needs, as well as what would be required at other levels of advancement. The framework was extensively used across the four UK countries by those within, or leading, public health teams to aid recruitment and development and by those running public health courses to ensure that they were pitched at the right level and covered the required content (Carlson, 2008; Wright et al, 2008). A major weakness of the framework, however, was its failure to be formally taken up by the DH (and thereby employing organisations) as a way of recognising competency across the whole public health workforce. Because of this, it was not fully embedded within career structures and linked to required training and development for, particularly, specific roles or grades of the public health practitioner workforce.

Figure 7.1: The 'PHRUBIK' cube

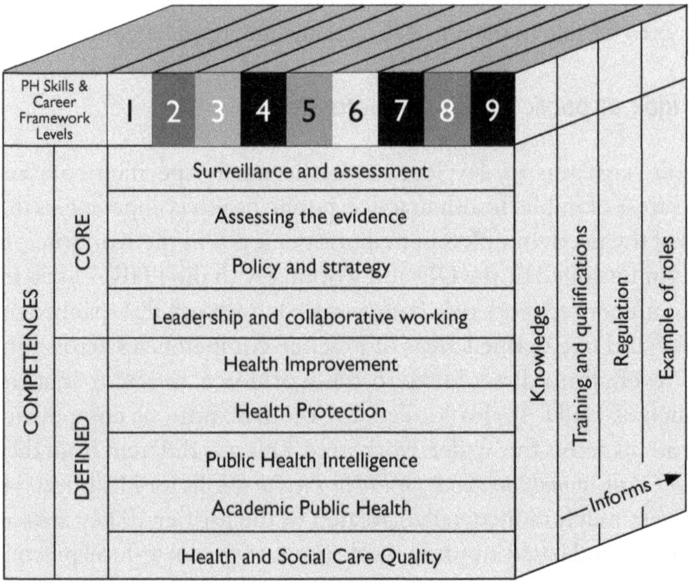

Note: PHRUBIK cube - a pun on Rubik's cube

Source: www.phorcast.org.uk (accessed 14 January 2014). See also Skills for Health (2008).

Health trainers – a new public health workforce

The *Choosing health* White Paper (DH, 2004b) was also used to announce the launch of a new programme, funded by the DH, to establish health trainers across the country. This new cadre of front-line public health workforce, trained in behaviour change, was to have a vital role in working with individuals to help them adopt healthier lifestyles: 'They will work with individuals to agree personalised health plans and overcome barriers to changes' (Bimpe et al, 2006). Funding was allocated initially to the most deprived 20% of geographical areas, which were designated to be spearheads for the initiative (Green, 2007). Health trainers were recruited from local communities to work with individuals in a variety of locations, including the NHS, prisons, post offices, the army, schools and libraries. Formal basic training and qualifications were provided. A qualitative review of health trainer programmes in two PCTs between 2007 and 2009 revealed satisfaction with the role and achievements of those health trainers and their managers interviewed, but some concern about where they fitted into overall service provision (Ball and Nasr, 2011). Following cuts to the DH public health development programme, 2011 was the last year of national funding, though many PCTs continued to commission this workforce at the local level.

Information on the breadth of public health careers and how to attain them

A further project funded by the DH public health workforce development team following the *Choosing health* White Paper (DH, 2004b) was the development of a UK public health careers website. This was in response to concerns about capacity following the 2006 health service reforms (DH, 2005) and the lack of an obvious source to find out about the range of public health careers and how to attain them. The website was developed by the PHRU working with East Midlands Healthcare Workforce Deanery, and was launched in April 2010.[223]

Initiatives that did not make progress

Other initiatives, such as the accurate defining and counting of the public health practitioner workforce, did not come to fruition. A

---

[223] See: www.phorcast.org.uk. From April 2013, the UK public health careers website has moved to Health Education England, along with the NHS Careers and Medical Careers websites.

national workshop in September 2008, hosted by the DH, to look at the feasibility of extending the current health service Electronic Staff Records to include a refined data collection, which would be more sensitive to the needs of public health and recognise the richness of disciplines comprising the practitioner workforce, did not lead to further work. The 2013 *Public health workforce strategy* picked up this issue (DH et al, 2013).

An unpublished review of academic public health carried out by Solutions for Public Health (SPH) for the DH in 2010 (Dunkley and Wright, 2010) reported on the long-standing issues of uncertainty of employment for non-medical public health researchers on a series of short-term contracts and lack of equality of opportunity and pay compared with the medical academic workforce.[224] Again, this issue, along with overall concern about the state of academic public health, medical and non-medical, was picked up in the 2013 *Public health workforce strategy* (DH et al, 2013) which promised further work led by Public Health England (PHE).

The Faculty of Public Health: a specialist professional body only or inclusive of practitioners? A strategic approach to practitioner recognition and development

The FPH had a long-standing interest in working with different public health professional organisations over developing a common approach to competency, not only for those organisations representing or regulating the workforce at specialist level (eg General Dental Council [GDC], College of Paediatrics and Child Health, and Faculty of Occupational Medicine), but also for those representing practitioner groups such as public health pharmacy and public health nursing.

From 2005, the FPH had a number of different strands of work under way relating to the development of the public health practitioner workforce. It set up its own practitioner development project in 2005, part funded by the DH, in the wake of the UKPHR-led work to prepare for registration of specialists in defined areas of practice and the forthcoming Skills for Health UK public health competency framework. Its newsletter for members in June 2006 (*Ph.com*, 2006), for example, had specific articles recognising the range of those working in public

---

[224] 'Academic public health in England', SPH, August 2010; personal archive of the authors.

---

health practitioner roles, including information and intelligence, public health nursing, health promotion, environmental health, and pharmacy. The FPH had already created a category of associate membership (for a small sum, anyone could subscribe and receive regular news updates) and wanted to consider whether it should set up formal practitioner membership at some stage and what this would entail if it did.

A working group was established to undertake further scoping work. Part of its remit was to consult with the national public health organisations and informal groups representing different contributions to public health (including environmental health, public health intelligence, health protection, nursing, health promotion, health psychologists, health services, public health academics and public health nutrition) over how practitioner competency could be formally recognised and the potential role of the FPH in this process as a possible standard-setting body for the whole of public health practice.[225] At the time, the FPH was the standard-setting body for specialists only. As stated earlier in this chapter, the only groups that had formal recognition and registration at practitioner level in public health were environmental health and public health nursing on a statutory basis and public health nutrition through voluntary regulation. There was a lack of clarity over whether practitioners needed to be regulated for public protection and whether registration and regulation would enhance personal and career development.

Another strand of work considered changes to the higher specialist training scheme. A formal Practitioner Committee was established at the FPH in October 2007, with a brief to consider whether prospective higher specialist training routes leading to registration at specialist level were needed for practitioners in the five defined areas of public health practice (health improvement, health intelligence, health and social care quality, health protection, and academic public health). Discussions were already under way across the national public health organisations over a strategic approach to the development of the whole practitioner workforce and these ran alongside the setting up of registration for defined specialists. There was also concern, in the interests of both public protection and career progression, to have recognition of practitioners at appropriate career points. Following agreement across national public health organisations in March 2006 to move to recognition of four core and five defined areas of public health practice, the FPH was also considering at this time whether its

---

[225] Paper to FPH board, February 2007; personal archive of the authors.

Part A examination should be offered in sections in diploma form to meet the needs of specific areas of practice.

In the event, the FPH moved away from consideration of practitioners to retain its role as a membership body and standard-setter for specialists only. Following a change of personnel within the DH, funding to support the FPH's practitioner development work ceased from 2008. The revision of the FPH's core curriculum did not include higher specialist training routes for defined areas of practice and the requirement for all trainees to demonstrate competency in all four core and five defined areas of practice was retained in order to qualify for the mandatory Certificate of Completion of Training (CCT). This subsequently left the UKPHR in some difficulties – as well as practitioners themselves – as its retrospective portfolio assessment route for defined specialists had been introduced in 2006 with the aspiration that, in future, there would be a prospective training route for defined specialists with equivalence to that for generalists.

The UK Public Health Register opens up its register to practitioners

The UKPHR started to work on the possibility of developing a regulatory framework for public health practitioners in 2006, following the *Choosing health* White Paper (DH, 2004b), and, with DH funding support, launched a major consultation exercise with the practitioner workforce from 2007. It used the UKPHSCF (Skills for Health, 2008) competencies as the basis for developing a draft set of standards for public health practitioners at graduate level in the workforce. A formal consultation took place in November 2008 on its proposals for retrospective recognition via portfolio assessment for practitioners (Somervaille, 2008). Standards were finalised and a process for retrospective recognition developed, which, because of the potentially large numbers seeking recognition, and to make it financially viable, was established as a devolved scheme using UKPHR-trained local assessors and verifiers of practitioner competency, with quality assurance of local schemes provided by the UKPHR.

According to the UK Public Health Careers website,[226] initially, both practitioner and advanced practitioner registration and regulation 'levels' were identified by the UKPHR as being needed to provide a proper career structure for public health practitioners. However, the Council

---

[226] Available at: http://www.phorcast.org.uk/page.php?page_id=278 (accessed September 2013).

for Healthcare Regulatory Excellence (CHRE), now the Professional Standards Authority for Health and Social Care (PSA)[227] advised that much of what is called 'advanced practice' represented an individual's career progression and should be recognised through professional accreditation rather than through regulation. The UKPHR decided, therefore, to progress with only a single (graduate) level of formal practitioner registration and regulation at that point.

DH funding support to the UKPHR for its practitioner work ceased from 2010. A further blow for the UKPHR was the conclusion of the DH-commissioned regulatory review on public health that the case for practitioner regulation was not proven (DH, 2010c). The UKPHR board decided, however, that there was sufficient demand to launch voluntary practitioner registration as a pilot programme from May 2011 and invited locally funded schemes to participate. Registration was only permitted for practitioners taking part in UKPHR-approved pilot schemes and the UKPHR instituted tight quality assurance. Early adopters were Wales and South Central England, where local development work in preparation for the opening of the register started in 2010. They were followed from 2011/12 by the South East Coast, West Midlands, Bristol and Glasgow and the Highlands in Scotland. A scheme for 12 practitioners in the South West and one across the 10 boroughs in North Central, North East Inner and Greater London started in 2013.

At September 2013, there were 95 practitioners registered with the UKPHR, with many more preparing for registration (from an estimated potential pool across the UK of 40,000). Since 2013, the UKPHR has been working on a programme to require Continuing Professional Development (CPD) for registered practitioners and intends, in time, to develop revalidation requirements.[228]

Some practitioners working not far below consultant level had been attracted to aim for defined specialist registration as the only formal route to progression open to them apart from the higher specialist training scheme. As one commentator from the UKPHR stated: 'some people had thrown themselves into defined specialist registration because there is nothing else'.[229] Similarly, a number of the early practitioner registrants with the UKPHR were working at levels well

[227] April 2014: UK Public Health Register's voluntary register of public health specialists and practitioners was accredited by the Professional Standards Authority for Health and Social Care [PSA] under the PSA's Accredited Voluntary Registers (AVR) scheme. Details can be accessed at: www.publichealthregister.org.uk/node/218
[228] Personal communication with UKPHR CEO, October 2013.
[229] Personal communication, 2013.

above the minimum (graduate) level required for registration, anxious to have some form of formal recognition.[230]

As yet, there is no employer requirement for practitioner regulation, apart from those who have to be statutorily regulated (eg environmental health officers and public health nurses). Practitioner regulation was not directly covered in the *Public health workforce strategy* (DH et al, 2013). The UKPHR chair, however, stated at a celebration of the first 10 years of the register on 4 September 2013 that, on the basis of the pilot schemes, it was aiming to launch a national programme for practitioner registration during 2014. It was in active discussion with Public Health England (PHE) over this, as a major employer (alongside local government) of the public health practitioner workforce since April 2013.

Recognising the value of the wider public health workforce

While the potential importance of the wider public health workforce had been recognised in *The report of the Chief Medical Officer's project to strengthen the public health function in England* (Donaldson, 2001) and by Derek Wanless (2002, 2004) in his 'fully engaged scenario', in reality, little had happened since then to turn that potential into practice. The problem then, as now, was not only identifying this more nebulous workforce, but also getting their engagement and changing practice on a large scale.

A project conducted in London in 2002 had attempted to map the wider workforce and ascertained that the total public health workforce in London, the majority of whom would comprise the wider workforce, potentially numbered up to a quarter of a million people from an enormously diverse range of occupations, who met the inclusion criteria for having the potential for improving the health of the community or population for which they worked (Sim et al, 2002). In keeping with the earlier CMO's project to strengthen the public health function (Donaldson, 2001), this mapping exercise recommended subdividing the wider workforce, for example: chief

---

[230] An interesting corollary has been the progression of dental public health, where the decision of the GDC was only to register and regulate qualified dentists at specialist level although the GDC does register dental practitioners (hygienists, dental nurses and therapists). This is possibly because dental public health is a very small specialty, and following recognition of competency with the Faculty of Public Health (FPH) at specialist level, a number of dental public health consultants had moved into generalist public health roles.

executives in local government and in the NHS who had a strategic role (who were described as 'key influencers' for health); experts and scientists from a range of disciplines, for example, toxicologists and traffic engineers ('technical experts'); clinicians and the hands-on workforce, such as social workers, who were working with users; and commissioners, business managers, service providers and audit/quality assurance staff, who use contracts, governance and audits to deliver and measure quality and outcomes.

Initiatives from 2006

The Head of Public Health Workforce Development at the DH in 2006 commented:[231] '*Choosing health* was the best opportunity to deliver change for the public health workforce and [it is] always important to build on whatever opportunities [are] offered.' She had been able to lead writing of the workforce chapter of *Choosing health* (DH, 2004b) and she could then peg initiatives to it. Slogans such as 'public health is everybody's business' gave credibility and legitimacy, and, with these, funding for specific initiatives. One of these initiatives was the Healthy Universities network, established in 2006 and continued with modest support from the higher education sector, with universities able to market themselves as healthy organisations.

A second initiative was the establishment of Teaching Public Health Networks (TPHNs).[232] In December 2005, the DH hosted a conference to launch these new networks, whose function would be to extend knowledge and skills to large numbers of people who would become identified members of the wider public health workforce. The broad objective was to boost teaching capacity in a range of educational institutions to ensure that public health skills would be disseminated among a diverse workforce. The TPHNs were established with agreed key deliverables, including an increase in teaching capacity and increases in the numbers of participants in a range of relevant courses provided by colleges of further education and institutions of higher education. The intention here was to build capacity on a large scale through participation in existing mainstream educational courses.

The FPH newsletter (*Ph.com*) in June 2006 was devoted to the concept of the inclusive public health workforce, although no one really had an understanding of how this was to be achieved. The TPHNs would set

---

[231] Personal communication, 2013.

[232] The TPHNs were called 'teaching' to distinguish them from 'research', which was the CMO's prerogative.

out to introduce pilot initiatives for the training and development of the wider workforce with a view to further roll-out if successful.

The DH invited expressions of interest in setting up TPHNs following the consultation meeting in December 2005. The outcome of this exercise was a skewed distribution of interest around the country, so the DH revisited its invitation and made an expectation that there would be one TPHN in each of the NHS regions to ensure a more equitable distribution of both infrastructure and outputs. After a further round of proposals to the DH, nine TPHNs were approved, covering the whole of England. Funding was distributed pragmatically, using a combination of an evaluation of the content of the proposals and the population base. The TPHNs were established during late 2006 through 2007 (Sim, 2007).

Each TPHN was invited to take a lead interest in a particular topic or part of the workforce, or both. The model adopted was similar to that of the Public Health Observatories, although the TPHNs lacked the stability of the Observatories, which enjoyed substantial personal support and patronage from the CMO, and a stable level of funding. Nevertheless, useful work was undertaken. In London, for example, at the first meeting of the TPHN Steering Group, there was consensus that the priority should be on building capacity in the third (voluntary) sector – thus, this became a lead area for London's TPHN, and, subsequently, as a result of the award of additional grant funding, a second lead area was added, that of childhood obesity. The London TPHN work with the third sector led to a feasibility study for creating a Health Passport for Health and Wellbeing, a concept that was revived by the DH in 2013 for the public health workforce in its strategy for the public health workforce (DH, 2013). The South West TPHN led on building capacity in relation to the built environment, and the South Coast led on incorporating public health into teacher training. The outputs of the TPHNs, many of which were innovative and original, were shared through its informal Association of Teaching Public Health Networks (ATPHN) and captured on the association's website (no longer active).

An early task of the TPHNs was to map existing educational provision for the wider public health workforce, but this became an enormous task, with hundreds of courses in further and higher education having at least some content that was relevant to public health, though few used the conventional terminology of public health. Nevertheless, networks were able to review some course content, and the importance of the UKPHSCF, published in 2008 by Skills for Health, to wider workforce development should not be underestimated. It provided, for the first time, the concept of core competencies needed by anyone working in any field at any level in public health and was used extensively by TPHNs for course mapping and informing new course development.

In 2007, the potential role of the wider public health workforce was considered in an international context by Sim et al (2007) in the *Bulletin of the World Health Organisation*. They described different ways for building capacity in public health, recognising the great size of the wider workforce and that many may be in third sector organisations, as well as in a variety of independent sector organisations. They highlighted the roles played by the leisure sector, for example, in addition to those working in health and social care, education, and housing and planning departments. The authors called for ways that are more open and inclusive of people from a wide range of educational and occupational backgrounds not previously the target of public health training.

The wider workforce in the reformed National Health Service and public health systems

The Marmot (2010) review on health inequalities, *Fair society, healthy lives*, issued in February 2010, highlighted the social gradient of health, whereby the lower one's social and economic status, the poorer one's health. He called for action across all the social determinants of health, including education, employment, income, home and community, and provided new impetus for looking at the contributions to the delivery of health outcomes across many workforces.[233]

Following the English health system reforms in 2013,[234] responsibility for development of the wider public health workforce rests across Health Education England (HEE) and its constituent Local Education and Training Boards (LETBs), PHE, and individual local authorities.[235] It is in the interests of hospital trusts, sitting on these new LETBs, to invest in promoting public health awareness in their own workforces not only to enhance their own staff's health, but to provide information for their one-to-one contacts with patients. Local authorities may choose to develop the wider workforce. There is no mandatory requirement to do so, although one aim in moving NHS public health teams into upper-tier local authorities is to help them focus more holistically on their public health outcomes. Health and Wellbeing Boards – the newly

---

[233] One response to the Marmot review was the Coalition government's pledge in February 2011 to increase the number of health visitors to 4,200 by 2015 (DH, 2011, p 4) to provide renewed focus on ensuring all families have a positive start.

[234] For details on the reformed structures, see Chapter Eight.

[235] For details on the reformed structures, see Chapter Eight.

appointed statutory bodies set up as local authority committees and normally chaired by a local councillor – with local strategic oversight of health in its widest sense, may well play a part in future. Senior officers from PHE have indicated their recognition of the importance of the wider workforce and commitment to its development.

Meanwhile, initiatives that began prior to the reforms were embedded to varying extents across the country. The NHS Future Forum set out clearly the role of the NHS in the promotion of health in it summary report (Field, 2012, p 8):

> Firstly, we must support the NHS to use every contact with patients and the public to help them maintain and improve their physical and mental health and wellbeing, including those already living with a condition. Each day, GPs [General Practitioners] and practice nurses see over 800,000 people and dentists see over 250,000 NHS patients. There are 31,000 NHS sight tests, while approximately 1.6 million people visit a pharmacy. Secondly, we must help the NHS workforce to improve their own health and act as role models for their patients and communities. And finally, we must embed the prevention of poor health and promotion of healthy living into the NHS's day-to-day business.

'Making every contact count' (MECC), whereby each encounter by a health care professional with a patient or service user would include a health promotion element, was subsequently adopted by a number of SHAs and a number of products were produced (including a tool kit in the East Midlands SHA[236] and a lifestyle, behaviour change competency framework in the Northern and Yorkshire SHA[237]), but implementation was not national and has not been monitored. Unless individual Clinical Commissioning Groups adopt it and/or choose to performance manage providers in this area of delivery, it may be impossible to evaluate the extent of its impact. What we do know from evaluation of projects that have been undertaken is that the methodology is sound, and that MECC has considerable potential for changing staff attitudes in relation to promoting health-enhancing behaviour among members of the general public coming into contact

---

[236] See: http://www.midlandsandeast.nhs.uk/OurAmbitions/Everycontactcounts.aspx (accessed September 2013).

[237] See: http://chain.ulcc.ac.uk/chain/documents/competenceframeworkintro.pdf (accessed April 2014)

---

with services (Nelson et al, 2013). The current distribution and reach of MECC remains unknown.

In the reformed health structures, HEE is responsible for development and training of the NHS workforce, which includes many members of the wider public health workforce. At the time of writing, it is unclear how the responsibilities of PHE and HEE will converge, but it is conceivable and, indeed necessary, that both of these new national agencies will collaborate to take the development of the wider public health workforce seriously.

What was achieved

- A focus on competency and development for the practitioner workforce.
- New skills and approaches in changing lifestyle behaviour.
- Some underpinning foundations for practitioner development in a common framework of competency for the whole of the public health workforce and bringing together information on the breadth of public health careers into one place.

Key learning points

- Importance of DH policy backing and funding to pump-prime initiatives.
- Importance of public health organisations working together to progress development.
- Importance of recognition of public health practice at different levels, which is independent of employing organisation.
- A recognised competency framework is the foundation for bringing together a disparate workforce and also providing a common language for accepted and acceptable practice.

EIGHT

Where we are now? The new public health system in England from April 2013

Introduction

The public health system in England is now radically different from all other decades that have been reported on so far in this book.

This chapter:

- outlines the changes to the public health and health systems in England, implemented from 1 April 2013;
- discusses their potential impact on the workforce; and
- considers the new public health workforce strategy and what the future holds for multidisciplinary public health development stemming from this.

New public health system for England from 2013

The Coalition government came to power in May 2010 with an agenda for radical reform of both the health service and the public health system. Driving forces were the stated intention to focus on outcomes rather than targets, increase choice and competition, give greater control to local clinicians, and ensure transparency of data. For public health, the aims were to give local communities greater control over public health budgets and to ensure that General Practitioners (GPs) were more engaged in the prevention agenda and tackling health inequalities. Despite the desire to reduce the overall size of the state sector, implementation has entailed considerable change and upheaval in both health service and public health administration and the creation of an extremely complex new system with a substantial number of new public sector organisations.

The reforms came into operation on 1 April 2013. The National Health Service (NHS) White Paper proposals (DH, 2010a) changed the structure for the commissioning of health care and thereby substantially increased GP engagement in commissioning. The 152 Primary Care

Trusts (PCTs), previously responsible for commissioning the whole of health care, and 10 Strategic Health Authorities (SHAs), providing performance oversight, were disbanded and replaced by a system of over 200 GP-led Clinical Commissioning Groups (CCGs). The latter were to be charged with commissioning the bulk of secondary care health services, working within and supported by a new structure called NHS England (also known as the NHS Commissioning Board), a Special Health Authority with a budget of £80 billion and operating as a single system through 27 Area Teams (ATs) across the country.[238]

Healthy lives, healthy people (DH, 2010b), the public health White Paper issued five months later, restructured the public health workforce and set up two principal arrangements for the future employment of the public health workforce: as part of either a new national civil service public health agency, Public Health England (PHE), or within (upper-tier[239]) local government.

These two changes marked a major departure for the public health workforce. Apart from those public health staff working in provider organisations, for example, staff delivering smoking cessation or screening programmes or those based in primary care, such as health visitors, very few core public health staff, and hardly any public health specialists, were to be directly employed within the health service.

Both White Papers were backed by outcomes frameworks, one for the NHS (DH, 2010d) and one for public health (DH, 2012a). A *Public health workforce strategy* for England was issued in 2013 (DH et al, 2013).

The White Papers were translated into the NHS and Social Care Bill, which was eventually enacted in April 2012 (as the NHS and Social Care Act 2012) after significant parliamentary and public debate and revision, but these main structural changes were retained.

Figure 8.1 sets out the new public health system. It is complex and multifaceted. From 1 April 2013, the professional specialist and practitioner public health workforce is principally employed either by PHE or by upper-tier councils.

The Department of Health

Funding for the health service and into public health is via an annual vote in Parliament and is channelled to the service through

---

[238] The King's Fund has an animated video on the new NHS, 'An alternative guide to the new NHS in England'. Available at: http://www.kingsfund.org.uk/projects/nhs-65/alternative-guide-new-nhs-england (accessed March 2014).

[239] County councils, unitary authorities or metropolitan boroughs.

Figure 8.1: The public health system in England with effect from 1 April 2013

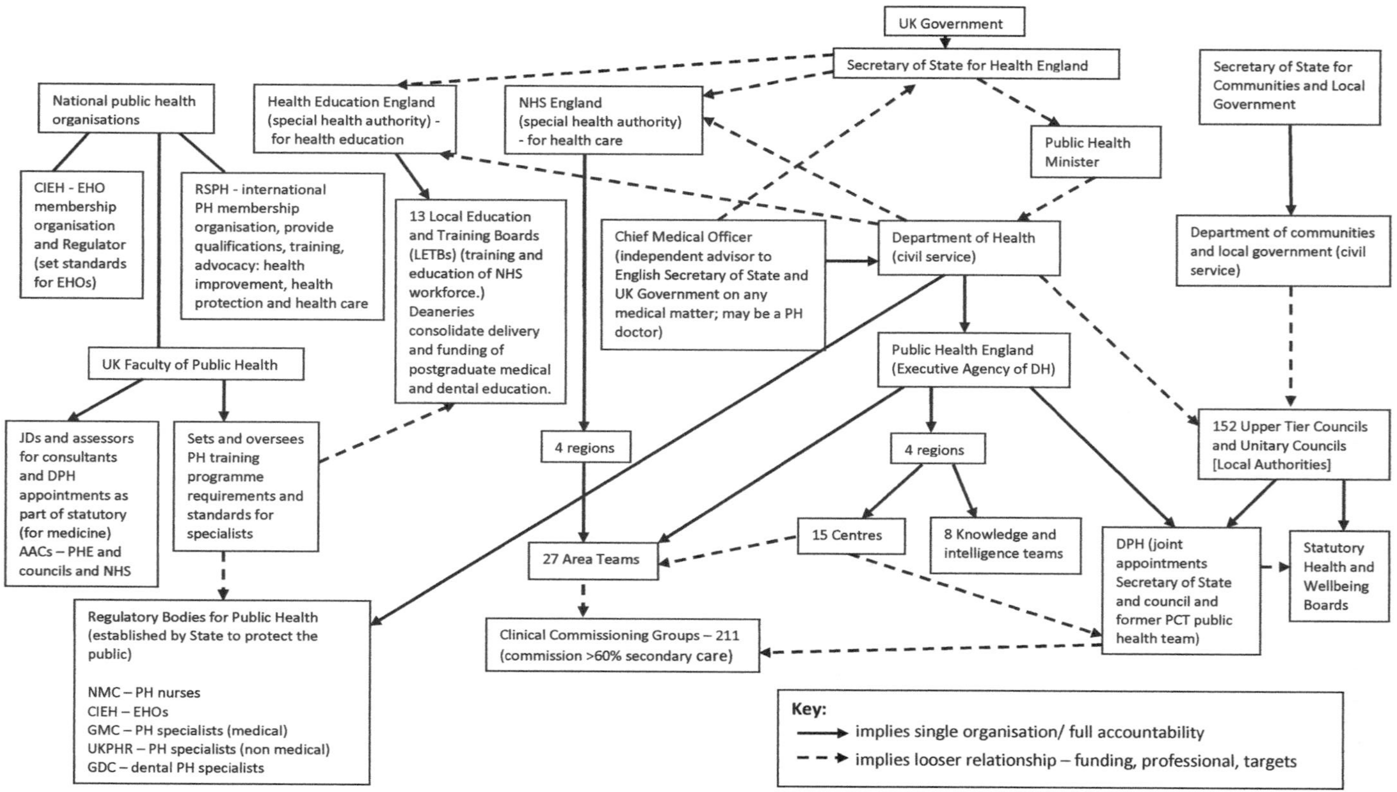

the Department of Health (DH). The DH remains the government department responsible for strategy, policy and funding for health and health care. Some changes have been made, however, in its responsibilities and those of its ministers.

Changes in responsibilites within the DH

The Secretary of State for Health, as a government minister, is responsible for:

- oversight of NHS delivery and performance;
- implementation of reform;
- overall financial control; and
- relationships with NHS England and Monitor (sector regulator for health care).

The Minister for Public Health reports to the Secretary of State and has specific responsibilities for:

- preventing avoidable mortality;
- the relationship with PHE and with the public health system;
- health protection and improvement; and
- vaccination.

The focus of the DH, which still employs over 2,000 civil servant staff, is now less on delivery and more on strategy, policy and outcomes. Its role is to set national policies for health and care and pursue the Secretary of State's statutory duties, including improving service quality, reducing inequalities, improving efficiencies and protecting and improving the public's health. As stated on its website:[240]

> We lead across health and care by creating national policies and legislation, providing the long-term vision and ambition to meet current and future challenges, putting health and care at the heart of Government; we support the integrity of the system by providing funding, assuring the delivery and continuity of services and accounting to Parliament in a way that represents the best interests of the patient, public and taxpayer.

The DH is structured under a permanent secretary with five director generals (one of whom is for public health) and the Chief Medical

---

[240] Available at: www.dh.gov.uk (accessed August 2013).

Officer (CMO) for England. It has a departmental board and executive board.

It supports the public health system through its arm's-length executive agency, PHE, and by providing ring-fenced funding (£5.4 billion for the first two years at least) to upper-tier councils to commission specified public health programmes through local government and also funding to NHS England (£2.2 billion) to commission specific public health programmes (such as prison health and screening) through its ATs. It produced the *Public health workforce strategy* (DH et al, 2013) in April 2013 and is expected to consult upon and oversee implementation of appropriate statutory arrangements for the regulation of non-medical specialists in public health.

The CMO is the independent adviser to the Secretary of State and the UK government on all medical matters, as well as being the Chief Scientific Adviser to the DH. He/she supports the government to ensure that decisions on health and social care are based on the most up-to-date and reliable research evidence. The post may be, but is not always, held by a public health doctor.

Public Health England

PHE, an arm's-length civil service agency employing over 5,500 staff, with a budget from 2013 of £800 million, brought together: staff from the former Health Protection Agency (HPA); staff working on national health data management and intelligence functions (such as the Public Health Observatories and cancer registries), as well as dental public health consultants; public health staff involved in the commissioning and quality assuring of screening programmes; and those providing public health advice to some as aspects of highly specialised tertiary services commissioning. Like NHS England, it has a nationwide single operating model.

Its overall remit is to improve health and reduce inequalities by supporting the delivery of the Public Health Outcomes Framework (increased healthy life expectancy and reduced differences in life expectancy and healthy life expectancy between communities) (DH, 2012a). It will also play a key role in, and have specific posts dedicated to, public health workforce and development.

According to its website,[241] as the expert voice in health protection and improvement, PHE's responsibilities are:

---

[241] Available at: http://www.gov.uk/government/organisations/public-health-england (accessed August 2013).

- making the public healthier by encouraging discussions, advising government and supporting action by local government, the NHS and other people and organisations
- supporting the public so they can protect and improve their own health
- protecting the nation's health through the national health protection service, and preparing for public health emergencies
- sharing our information and expertise with local authorities, industry and the NHS, to help them make improvements in the public's health
- researching, collecting and analysing data to improve our understanding of health and come up with answers to public health problems
- reporting on improvements in the public's health so everyone can understand the challenge and the next steps
- helping local authorities and the NHS to develop the public health system and its specialist workforce.

PHE is structured into 10 directorates under the Chief Executive Officer (CEO). Their directors, as well as the regional directors, sit on the executive, which has an advisory board. PHE has incorporated the UK National Screening Committee and the senior dental public health workforce.[242]

Like NHS England, the new agency operates as a single organisation, working on a distributed model through four regional teams, 15 local centres and eight knowledge and intelligence teams. Some staff are posted to NHS England ATs to provide public health expertise to specific commissioning functions, such as specialised services and screening programmes.

The role of the four regions, which mirror those for NHS England – North, South, Midlands and East of England, and London – is described by PHE on its website as follows:

- to manage strategic discussions with partners
- give professional support and leadership to the public health system including jointly appointing Directors of Public Health
- see that PHE centres provide consistently high-quality services, address local needs and priorities and contribute to improving local health
- make sure the region has a national emergency planning, resilience and response strategy.

---

[242] PHE has a Director of Dental Public Health. The Chief Dental Officer and Deputy Chief Dental Officer sit in NHS England.

The 15 centres are described as the 'front door' for most of PHE's local services across health improvement, health care public health and health protection by giving local government access to specialised support and advice through the Directors of Public Health (DsPH). The intention is that these centres work closely with NHS England, developing and supporting the people who work in public health and managing PHE's relationship with Local Education and Training Boards (LETBs). London has a modified structure, enabling it to function as an integrated region and centre.

The eight knowledge and intelligence teams (KITs) provide a service to local authorities and other partners in the public health system, including Health and Wellbeing Boards. The teams include staff and functions from the former Cancer Intelligence Units, Drug Treatment Monitoring Units and Public Health Observatories.

Local government

Upper-tier local government authorities (county councils, metropolitan boroughs and unitary authorities) were given new statutory responsibilities for public health under the Health and Social Care Act 2012. These 152 upper-tier authorities must: (a) establish Health and Wellbeing Boards with a local strategic role to underpin local health and social care commissioning; (b) commission specific local public health programmes, such as NHS health checks, sexual health services, the National Child Measurement Programme and Healthy Child Programme (5–19);[243] (c) protect the health of the population; and (d) provide public health advice to the local health service, especially the local CCGs. To carry out these additional functions, these councils across England were allocated two-year ring-fenced funding from April 2013 of £5.4 billion from the DH. To support delivery of the new responsibilities, public health staff from the former NHS PCTs, including DsPH (formally, a joint appointment between the local authority and secretary of state), were transferred into local government employment from 1 April 2013.

Health care public health

A major omission in the original White Papers in 2010 (DH, 2010a, 2010b) was consideration of the third domain of public health – health

---

[243] Early years services for child health commissioned by NHS England (Healthy Child Programme [0–5]).

and social care quality – causing concern about how specialist advice would be accessed by the NHS and bringing added uncertainty for any staff working in that sphere of public health at the time.

It was not clear from the two White Papers how NHS commissioning would, in future, receive local public health advice on clinical and cost-effectiveness, population data interpretation, and public health input to health service reconfiguration. From late 2011 onwards, an uneasy compromise model emerged whereby CCG public health support was to come from a mandatory 'core offer' from upper-tier local authorities, using their incoming NHS public health staff to deliver this. The content of the 'core offer' was not specified nationally, however, and, anecdotally, it has been applied variably in different places depending upon views within individual local councils, the availability of local public health skills and the capacity and local requirements of individual CCGs.

The transition

Implementation of the reforms was marked by a long transition period of nearly three years. In part, this was because of the complexity of the employment changes and the volume of staff across the country in health, and in public health, who were changing not only roles, but employers. Some public health specialist staff took voluntary redundancy or early retirement, as had happened in previous reorganisations. Another reason for the slow progress was because of natural resistance to change. According to Hunter:

> if you want to disturb the status quo it makes little sense to entrust the task to those who either consider themselves to be at risk or who stand to lose most from the changes. (Hunter, 2013, p1)

Earlier Hunter had commented that disruptive innovation was never likely to find favour among certain groups in public health, largely, though not exclusively, those with a clinical background – who, with few exceptions, are cautious, risk averse and have always been suspicious of local government. (Hunter, 2010)

There were perceived anxieties about the potential loss of independence for public health within both local government and the civil service public health agency. Hunter considers that the result may well have been a 'fudge' on both counts.

The public health *practitioner* workforce entered the transition, following the NHS and Public Health White Papers in 2010, uncertain about its future status and opportunities. Those NHS-employed staff working within PCTs or SHAs were destined either for local authority health improvement work or for the civil service as part of the new national agency, PHE, working chiefly in health improvement, health protection or health intelligence. In any event, they would be leaving the NHS. Although government policy in the 2000s had encouraged public health delivery through joint working between the health service and local government, public health practitioners had been employed principally within the health service.

Tensions between medical and non-medical public health staff re-emerged over employment opportunities and tensions also arose between national public health organisations over the voice for public health. Despite retirements, vacancies and the resultant public health workforce shortages, very few new consultant appointments were advertised during the transition, causing particular anxieties over employment opportunities for those completing, or just about to complete, their higher specialist training, as well as real challenges for maintaining safe public health delivery during the transition, including, in particular, during the period of the London 2012 Olympics and Paralympics (Sim, 2012).

And the future, one year after implementation

Because of the extremely complex nature of the changes introduced by the Coalition government, an extended period of settling in has been required for the new systems. There has been no formal evaluation published to date on progress of either the new health care commissioning or public health systems. However, two House of Commons select committees looked at the impact of changes in the run-up to implementation.

The Parliamentary Health Select Committee, in its 12th Report, published on 19 October 2011,[244] commented on specific changes, including the fact that the secretary of state for health would, for the first time, be under an explicit statutory duty to take appropriate steps to protect the public from dangers to health. The report criticised the lack of a statutory duty on local authorities to address health inequalities in discharging their public health function. Alongside

---

[244] Available at: www.publications.parliament.uk/pa/cm201012/cmselect/ cmhealth/1048/104802.htm (accessed December 2013).

this, they foresaw risks from ring-fencing funding to upper-tier local councils, fearing that they would see only this budget as relevant to public health and thereby miss the opportunities afforded by these reforms to change local government's perspective on health and public health. They were concerned that the mandated 'core offer' of public health advice to CCGs and the health service from local government would be insufficient. They felt that DsPH should be members of each CCG. They also recommended that all DPH applicants be subject to a statutory appointments process, including an Advisory Appointments Committee approved by the FPH. An equally major concern was the potential fragmentation of provision of public health services across local government, NHS England and PHE.

The House of Commons Communities and Local Government Select Committee looked at the role of local authorities in health issues in its eighth report of the 2012/13 session, published on 27 March 2013, just before the new system was implemented.[245] They had concerns about the new Health and Wellbeing Board: 'with few powers and no budgets to commission services themselves, they will have to display leadership, build relationships and use their influence locally to turn their health and wellbeing strategies into reality'. They were also not convinced that health emergencies were fully covered in the new arrangements, querying who would be in charge locally in the event of an emergency: 'the Government needs to set out the lines of responsibility between (local) organisations and confirm that PHE will have sufficient staff in its local teams to deal with contingencies'. Regarding DsPH, the Committee expressed concerns about their advice being heard, in that they might not report directly to local authority CEOs. They also queried their conflicting responsibilities: both sitting on and policing the Health and Wellbeing Boards.

These reforms do present new opportunities for public health, not least in being able to exert a positive influence for health both at the national level, with the creation, for the first time, of a potentially powerful public health agency, and at the local level, within local authorities and CCGs. Some interesting possibilities, as well as risks, challenges and unintended consequences, do arise, therefore, from the changes to and the potential impact on the public health system in England. We speculate on these.

---

[245] Available at: www.publications.parliament/uk/pa/cm201213/cmselect/cmcomloc/694/694vw.pdf (accessed December 2013).

Public Health England: the leading voice for public health?

Will PHE, because of its size and status, be seen as the employer of choice for public health? It will certainly have a major role in influencing strategy and policy at the centre, although there are questions, because of its civil service status, over how independent it can be in reality. If not PHE, will the advocacy role for public health be left to non-governmental national public health organisations? It is too early to state the full impact on the public health system of this new agency. Because of its size and status, there is no doubt that it will be a major player. The concerns of some specialists that local government will not respect their consultant status may provide a further driver for specialists, perhaps doctors especially, to seek employment in PHE.

A framework agreement between the DH and PHE was issued in November 2013,[246] which states:

> the Government's decision to establish PHE as an Executive Agency was driven by the need to provide the operational autonomy necessary for its scientific and professional work to be, and to be seen as, independent from DH. PHE's credibility will be based on its expertise, underpinned by its freedom to set out the evidence, science and professional public health advice it presents without fear or favour.

There are still risks, however. PHE will be 'closer' to the DH than the HPA, which was an arm's-length body. It will be harder, therefore, to retain independence. One interviewee referred to PHE as the 'nationalisation of public health'.[247]

The majority of staff entering PHE came from the HPA and their systems appear to have prevailed to a large extent in the new organisation. Incoming intelligence functions are numerically much smaller and come from a variety of small units, some from within the NHS but others from the university sector. It remains to be seen how effective and efficient the single operating model for PHE will be and whether it will lead to additional bureaucracy. It is likely to lead to a less participative style of delivery, although the PHE centres and KITs will need to liaise closely with local government and the local health system. The risk is that health protection issues will dominate the agenda.

---

[246] 'Framework agreement between the DH and Public Health England', PHE publications Gateway Number 2013234, 15 November 2013.

[247] Personal communication, 2013.

A recent Witness Seminar (Snow et al, 2013), held to capture the history of the HPA, provides some valuable insights into establishment issues and also into the potential for PHE, particularly because staff from the HPA are by far the largest group within PHE. As we have seen in Chapter Three, the HPA was established to raise the standards of the health protection services and ensure consistency across the country. It brought together into a single body people from 80 organisations across 140 locations, with different terms and conditions of service, IT systems, cultures, and histories. Staff reactions ranged from enthusiasm to hostility. Its first CEO described it as a 'painful birth'. There were some clear lessons from the process, particularly over the importance of developing a shared culture and giving emphasis to this rather than to structures and systems. Attendees at the Witness Seminar considered that the HPA's successes included having a well-known and trusted brand, high-calibre scientific expertise, and an ability to provide a joined-up response to public health events from local to national levels. Those in PHE will no doubt wish to build upon these strengths.

One of the major issues for the HPA was the creation of 'parallel hierarchies' between the HPA and NHS and, in particular, a confused and sometimes hostile relationship with local DsPH, some of whom had resented the transfer of consultant expertise into the HPA. The current relationship between local authority DsPH and directors within the PHE centres is unclear, and, as revealed earlier, in the parliamentary committee reports, there are still anxieties about accountabilities.

Employing senior public health professionals within local government to facilitate the realisation of health improvement opportunities?

Employing senior public health professionals within local government provides an opportunity for them to have influence across the whole council agenda. There are real opportunities for former NHS staff leading on health improvement to move into a variety of senior positions in local government as they evolve into more public health-facing organisations. Whereas there has been considerable support for local government having restored public health responsibilities, one risk is that some of the incoming former NHS public health staff are seen as just too expensive to justify their employment, once the financial ring-fence has expired, a risk that is accentuated at this time of austerity. In the longer term, salaries are likely to be lower than in the health service. Since senior medical salaries in the NHS have historically been higher than for other professions, a substantial concern is that the public health workforce employed within local government will become, over time, principally non-medical, with the potential of the 'downgrading' of both status and salaries.

Although the Agenda for Change job profiles for the public health workforce have been translated into local government profiles, salary scales vary greatly across the country and use of the profiles is not mandatory. Local authorities have considerable freedom over who they appoint and on what terms. There is, in particular, no statutory requirement to hold Advisory Appointment Committees for any staff outside the NHS.

A further concern is how public health doctors will be perceived within the medical workforce when once again employed by local government. After all, it took about 15 years for them to be accepted as equals within the health service medical workforce when they transferred to NHS employment in 1974. There are anxieties, too, that new medical recruits into public health specialist training may not wish to have careers in local government rather than the NHS in which they have been working since qualification. As well as salary, there will be implications for pensions and other aspects of employment that have yet to be fully understood.

Sustainability of public health advice into the National Health Service?

There remains uncertainty over how public health advice (around evidence base, clinical and cost-effectiveness, demand management, and service redesign) into the whole of the NHS will be acquired. The model of outsourcing a small cadre of public health professionals from PHE to NHS England ATs to cover specialised areas such as screening, immunisation and offender health provides a partial resolution. The sustainability of the model whereby local authority public health departments provide advice to CCGs is uncertain and capacity is scarce. The risk to sustainability will increase if fewer public health doctors who have expertise in health care public health, are employed within local government in the future. Some progressive GP training programmes have introduced public health modules, which, in time, may help to introduce some public health competencies into CCGs, but the Royal College of General Practitioners (RCGP) does not yet require such content in its national curriculum.

A changing Director of Public Health role?

Some commentators have suggested that these reforms are turning back the clock to 1974, the last time senior public health professionals were embedded within local government structures. The role of today's local authority DPH is rather different from that of the former, until 1974, Medical Officer of Health (MOH). Status within local government tends to be linked to size of departmental budgets and numbers of staff, and, while there are exceptions, most DsPH will not be running large departments or be responsible for large budgets in local government terms. They will, however, be expected to use their own, and their team's, skills, as well as the new mandatory public health requirements placed on local government, to influence health commissioning and planning across the whole organisation.

The local authority DPH role has oversight of the three domains of public health (and thereby maintains a unique position in public health in doing this). The role calls for new skills in influencing and negotiating within local government, although, in some areas, public health represents a relatively small department and budget and the DPH is not always directly accountable to the local authority CEO. It is not clear whether the DPH will be able to retain their independence as part of a democratically run organisation, and what this will mean in practice, nor how shared accountability to the secretary of state and to the local authority will actually play out in practice: as we have seen, the relationship between the local authority DPH and the local PHE Centre DPH remains unclear.

It is already apparent that there is considerable variability around the country in the structure of public health departments in local government and in the DPH role description – as one interviewee called it, 'postcode public health'.[248]

In some authorities, DsPH are located within Adult Social Care Directorates reporting to the Director of Adult Social Care and not the CEO. It is not clear whether this approach is more prevalent within county councils rather than unitary authorities. County council functions include social services, education and planning, whereas unitary authority functions include housing, trading standards, recreation and environmental health. Placing public health is, therefore, more likely to be difficult within county councils than within unitary authorities whose functions are much closer to traditional public health. Some commentators have suggested, therefore, that the policy

---

[248] Personal communication, 2013.

is urban-centric and may be less suited to the structures within shire counties (which more often have county councils). Adult social care, after all, reflects a small percentage of the population, whereas public health aims to address the needs of the whole population.

A few DsPH already have substantial departments well beyond public health and including environmental health and adult social care. According to Gamsu:[249]

> what we have here is a bit of a two way street. Some local authorities have clearly been impressed by the skills and experience of their Director of Public Health and considered that this means that they should also take on the adult social care portfolio. While others have been more impressed by what the adult social care profession has to offer and gone down that route.

In at least one authority, the role of DPH has gone to the Director of Adult Social Care (without public health qualifications), against FPH professional advice,[250] although PHE is working with such councils to ensure that suitable DPH advice is also available.[251] Some smaller unitary authorities, including those in London, have consultants in public health and teams, and an overarching DPH spanning a number of local authorities.

Apart from having a statutory DPH role, councils have complete freedom over the local structure for absorbing public health and there is considerable variability. Under a Freedom of Information Request, the FPH obtained information in August 2013 from all 156 local authorities in England[252] that 58 operated a stand-alone directorate. In some authorities, public health staff have been distributed across different council departments.

The Association of Directors of Public Health (ADsPH) survey of the transition in England six months on, published in January 2014,[253] raised concerns not only about the number of DPH posts that were vacant or

---

[249] Available at: http://localdemocracyandhealth.com (accessed December 2013).

[250] Within the NHS, it was easier to ensure that senior (consultant-level) appointments followed the professional guidance and process. It is less possible to enforce this in local government.

[251] Letter from the Chief Operating Officer for PHE 12 August 2013 to the FPH, Association of Directors of Public Health, UKPHR, UK Public Health Association, Royal Society for Public Health, British Medical Association; personal archive of the authors.

[252] Email communication, 13 December 2012; personal archive of the authors.

[253] Personal archive of the authors.

had interim/acting arrangements, but also about succession planning in the face of consultant vacancies and consultants gaining sufficient experience to provide the next generation of local authority DsPH.

Changing requirements for public health skills and a new kind of public health workforce?

It is not clear what the new structures and requirements will mean for the skills needed in future by the professional public health workforce. It is likely from the structures now in place that the public health workforce is more likely to work in specific areas of practice and not generically across the domains of public health – for example, in local government, it seems likely that public health departments will focus principally on delivering health improvement to the population, and in PHE, principally on health intelligence and health protection functions. It is not clear how easy it will be for staff to move around the system in future. Different settings will also require different skills and different approaches. Working in local government will require more participative, influencing and strategic roles, whereas much of PHE work will require public health staff with strong technical skills.

Some questions are already being asked over whether the service will need 'generalists', that is, public health professionals competent across all domains of public health practice, in the same way as in the past or whether the pattern of employment is leading to more narrowly defined areas of work, with consequent implications for future training and development. The current higher specialist training scheme does not, as yet, embrace this level of flexibility. The DPH may, indeed, be the only 'generalist' role remaining in the new structures, which begs the question of how future DsPH will be developed in the system. Even DsPH, however, do not have responsibilities spanning all public health functions in the reformed structure, for example, for screening and immunisation, as they would have had in the past.

It is clear that excellent and flexible leadership and management skills are needed to deliver these multifaceted public health roles in a very complex public health system, whether staff are in local government, PHE or outsourced to the health service. Those within local government have to learn to wield influence within a democratic system, and those within PHE, across the civil service and government, as well as across local health systems. Do we now need in future different skill sets for the challenges for different settings?

On a more positive note, these 2013 reforms also provide opportunities for a much wider range of staff to acquire baseline public health awareness and skills, such as planners, housing officers and social workers in local government, which was one of the intentions of the move of public health staff to local authorities.

Local authorities embracing their public health roles?

The Royal Society for Public Health (RSPH) commissioned a survey of public health teams working in local government, which was published in February 2014 (RSPH, 2014). Although optimistic overall, the survey revealed some anxieties, particularly where ring-fencing of public health monies were not always preserved for public health programmes and functions. Public health staff were concerned about decisions being taken on the basis of politics and not evidence, and felt that they needed additional influencing skills. The report acknowledges, however, that it is still early days following the transition.

System fragmentation leading to further change?

Because each local authority operates in a unique way, and CCGs have varying sizes, structures and priorities, there is no single approach to implementation of the new health system at the local level. This provides considerable flexibility and opportunity to do things differently – a 'natural' experiment. It could also mean that whereas some systems flourish, others may fare less well. Robust evaluation will be essential if we are to learn which models work best.

There is a real risk that an unintended consequence of the changes will be fragmentation of the public health system. Commissioning of some programmes is now, for example, spread across PHE, local authorities and CCGs. A simple example are the screening programmes funded by PHE, but commissioned via ATs within NHS England, supported by outsourced PHE public health staff and 'monitored' by public health teams within local government.

Public health staff are currently employed by a range of different organisations – civil service, local government and the NHS, as well as third and independent sector organisations – and, in time, this is likely to lead to very different structures, pay scales, titles and employment and career opportunities as each organisation starts to set its own direction for its staff. It is not clear what impact this will have on future generations of public health professionals or on attempts to develop a coherent public health workforce. It will be even harder to identify and count the workforce.

The main risk in fully implementing the reforms, however, may come from further destabilising change or further restructuring if there is a new government elected in 2015. The health system in England is rarely allowed enough time to bed down and deliver before being restructured.

The professional public health system

Health Education England (HEE) is now the oversight body for health care education and training for England, currently operating through 13 LETBs. Deaneries, responsible for coordinating delivery and funding for postgraduate medical and dental education, including the multidisciplinary public health training scheme, are subsumed within this structure. The FPH continues to set standards for specialist public health and public health training requirements for specialist status.

Regulation of public health specialists continues to be through the General Medical Council (GMC) for public health doctors, the General Dental Council (GDC) for public health dentists and the voluntary UK Public Health Register (UKPHR) for public health specialists from backgrounds other than medicine (although, in future, regulation of non-medical and dental specialists is anticipated to become statutory under the Health Care Professions Council [HCPC]). It is not clear, as yet, whether the UKPHR will continue to have any future role in the regulation of specialists. Neither is the long-term future for defined specialists determined, nor whether the UKPHR will continue to offer voluntary registration to this relatively small group of highly specialised public health workers. There is also no clarity regarding arrangements for revalidation of non-medical specialists if regulated by the HCPC.

Public health practitioners also continue to be regulated in a variety of ways: public health nurses statutorily with the Nursing and Midwifery Council (NMC); environmental health officers statutorily with the Chartered Institute of Environmental Health (CIEH); and some practitioners (still in relatively small numbers) voluntarily with the UKPHR. The great majority of practitioners are currently unregulated. The UKPHR has announced that, working with PHE, it aims to offer a national programme of practitioner registration from the spring of 2014.

The chair of the UKPHR stated on 3 September 2013 (at the meeting to celebrate 10 years of the register, held at the CIEH[254]) that the position of the UKPHR was to impress upon government the desirability of a single regulatory body for the whole of the public health

---

[254] Personal archive of the authors.

workforce – medical, non-medical (including dental) and practitioner. One advantage would be that this body would, at least, understand the whole of the public health context, which would not be the case if regulation for public health is a tiny part of a particular regulator's function. It would also facilitate career progression from practitioner through to specialist for those eligible to progress to specialist status. It is not clear, however, how feasible it would ever be to have a single regulatory agency for public health: it seems very likely that doctors and dentists, at least, would wish to retain their current medical and dental regulatory bodies. There is another view that too much emphasis has been placed on regulation to the detriment of looking at the whole of the public health workforce in a holistic way.

A new strategy for the public health workforce based on consultation with the workforce

A time of transition also presents opportunities for change. The DH, concerned about the impact of the reforms on the public health workforce and the need to have a workforce fit for the new purpose, issued a consultation paper in March 2012, co-branded with the Local Government Association, on the development of a workforce strategy for the new public health system (DH, 2012b). The consultation period was three months. This consultation was in the context of the new structure for the commissioning of health service education and training through HEE and the 12 LETBs, as described earlier.

The DH eventually published its *Public health workforce strategy* on 3 May 2013 (DH et al, 2013), along with a separate document summarising the comments received during the consultation period (DH, 2013). It should be borne in mind that the consultation took place at a time of maximum uncertainty for the workforce during the transition. The comments, however, are a good indication of the progress made in previous years in developing the whole of the public health workforce.

Categorising the public health workforce satisfactorily appeared to be a continuing issue. There was a fear in the consultation responses that being too specific about who is in, and who is out, of the public health workforce could mean exclusion of some valuable contributions to the public health endeavour. One suggestion in the consultation was to consider functions and who would be needed to deliver them rather than concentrating on specific professional groups. The inclusion of the 'wider public health workforce' in the categorisation was welcomed, although the strategy itself failed to pay attention to this large category and its potential contribution to public health.

There was a feeling that the development needs of the public health workforce moving into local government must be addressed. There were specific concerns about the disparity in opportunities between medical and non-medical staff within the academic public health workforce. The main comments were as follows (all quotes from DH, 2013):

1. There were continuing concerns about the disparity between opportunities for training and career enhancement between doctors and other groups: 'There is a strong view that non-medics and other related professional groups (for example nutritionists/dieticians) are not as well supported in their professional development as medically qualified colleagues and therefore fail to penetrate more senior management levels in public health' (p 12).
2. 'A significant number [of respondents] commented on the need for greater clarity (and communication) on training and development opportunities across all public health groups and career pathways' (p 13).
3. Many felt that the specialist–practitioner divide was unhelpful and simplistic and that a clear process for practitioners from a wide variety of areas to be enabled to access routes for training and development to public health consultant was needed. As one respondent stated: 'the portfolio route should have clearer learning and development competencies so staff can build up skills knowledge and expertise to enhance their role and work. This should be regardless of whether they ultimately submit a portfolio or not' (p 1).
4. There was some concern about how, in future, competency across the three domains of public health could be maintained within the new structures and how flexible the new system could be for the movement of staff across organisations. Some respondents were in favour of the creation of more joint posts, secondments and job shares (p 20).
5. The lack of joined-up leadership in public health and the lack of a united voice for the public health profession across organisations such as the CIEH, the RSPH, the FPH and the UKPHR was noted (p 21).

Responses to the public health workforce consultation: comments and concerns

The published strategy (DH et al, 2013) took a broad approach to the development of the workforce by aiming to strengthen the infrastructure. Specific programmes of work were set in train. The UK public health competency framework from Skills for Health (2008) was to be embedded, in an interactive form with clear guidance on use, within the UK Public Health Careers website, itself moving to HEE from April 2013. This followed a 'refresh' undertaken by the UK Public Health Careers website team, commissioned in 2012 by the UK Public Health Workforce Advisory Group and the DH to review and improve wider workforce competencies and improve ease of access and use of the whole framework for wide audiences.

A key recommendation, and one that was aimed at supporting progressive development of the whole workforce, was the proposed establishment of a web-based skills passport for public health. This followed earlier interest in one for the third sector and others, as we have seen in Chapter Seven, initiated by the London Teaching Public Health Network and Skills for Health in 2008/09, and also subsequent work that Skills for Health had undertaken to develop a skills passport for the whole of the NHS workforce. The passport for public health would allow for individual capture of qualifications and development in a systematic way, being common across the workforce and portable across different employing organisations, sectors and UK countries.

The following actions were also confirmed in the 2013 strategy (DH et al, 2013):

- Work was set in train to develop a minimum data set for the public health workforce.
- The DH would be consulting on proposals for statutory regulation of non-medically qualified specialists.
- Issues relating to specific practitioner groups were to be tackled – the non-clinical scientific workforce (moving from the HPA to PHE) linked to the 'Modernising scientific careers' programme (DH, 2010e), as well as the health intelligence workforce, principally within PHE, from April 2013.
- A separate initiative, led by PHE, would look at issues in academic public health.[255]

---

[255] The National School of Public Health was established in April 2012 as a partnership across eight academic centres and funded through the National Institute for Health Research for five years.

- The NHS Leadership Academy[256] would be charged with co-designing and developing leadership programmes.
- The FPH would be undertaking a curriculum refresh to ensure that training was fit for the public health skills required in the new system.
- The strategy announced that separate work would be undertaken to look at the needs of the local authority public health workforce.

What was not covered in the strategy

The strategy failed to cover some important issues:

- The future of practitioner regulation and advanced practitioner recognition.
- Outside of the training scheme, it was still not clear how career progression would work, which is a major concern of the practitioner workforce.
- The future of regulation and the status of defined specialists.
- There was no mention of the wider workforce or potential opportunities, using the new HEE and LETB structures, for ensuring that all health service and local government staff act to promote and facilitate healthy lifestyle behaviours in the course of their work.
- No strategic approach was taken to broadening the base of the public health workforce, such as including GPs, urban planners, housing officers and social workers, to reflect the new environments.
- Differentials in terms and conditions remain across the organisations employing public health staff or within the civil service arrangements within PHE.
- How existing good practice from promising local initiatives could be collected and shared more widely was not covered.

Some of these omissions may begin to be addressed as the new public health system takes shape, and as PHE starts to link strategically with NHS England, HEE and local government DsPHs. The risk is that PHE will focus on its own employees – each PHE region and centre will have leads for the public health workforce, for example – and not take full regard of those public health staff now within local authority structures, the NHS and other sectors. The issues relating to academic public health are very long-standing and currently remain unresolved. The strategy does not look fully, either, at the complex challenges faced

---

[256] See: www.leadershipacademy.nhs.uk (accessed January 2013).

by the public health workforce in the different settings in which it will operate and how to ensure that it will be fit for the new purpose.

What was achieved

- A new structure for the public health workforce in England from April 2013 with profound changes in roles and employment.
- A real opportunity for positive influence on health through the creation of an England-wide public health agency and placing public health staff at the heart of local government, but there are some risks in the system, particularly in providing public health advice to the NHS and NHS commissioning.
- An impetus, through the workforce strategy for public health, for relooking at the workforce and what is needed in the future to underpin delivery of better health outcomes.
- However, in the published *Public health workforce strategy* (DH et al, 2013), an opportunity was missed to recognise and develop the wider public health workforce.
- There remains lack of clarity concerning future arrangements for regulation of the workforce.

Key learning points

- Reforms marked by long and destabilising transition for the workforce with uncertainty over future employment.
- Considerable new opportunities for positively influencing health strategically.
- The local system will be marked by differential implementation.
- Risks in the system of silo working; loss of key skills and flexibility across domains and organisations.
- Commitment to work strategically to support the whole workforce in the new strategy, with further underpinning national structures.
- It will take time for the full implications and impact of the reforms to emerge.

NINE

Experience across the other UK countries

Introduction

The focus of this book has been on changes to the public health workforce in England. Because a number of the developments during the period covered by this book also applied to the public health workforce in the other three UK countries, it is useful to consider how each of them applied the changes and at what pace.

> **This chapter provides:**
>
> • brief information on how the public health workforce is structured in Wales, Scotland and Northern Ireland; and
> • an analysis as to how far each of the devolved administrations has progressed in introducing the changes to specialists and practitioners that have occurred in England since 1999.

England, with a population on census night 2011 of 53 million,[257] is by far the largest of the four UK countries. At the time of the census, Scotland had a population of 5.3 million, Wales 3.1 million and Northern Ireland 1.8 million.

Since the 1990s and the establishment of devolved administrations for Scotland, Northern Ireland and Wales, the health systems in the four countries have become increasingly divergent. Devolved powers for Scotland, Northern Ireland and Wales include responsibility for the organisation of health and social care. England is now the only one of the four countries, for example, to retain a full purchaser–provider split in health care. This has had an inevitable impact on the configuration of, and what has been required from, the public health workforce.[258]

---

[257] Office for National Statistics, 'Statistical bulletin 2011 census: population estimates for UK, 27 March 2011', released 17 December 2012.

[258] For detailed descriptions of each UK health system, see the UK Public Health Careers website. Available at: http://www.phorcast.org.uk/page.php?page_=1 (accessed September 2013).

Table 9.1: Summary of key similarities and differences in provision of health and social care across the UK countries

Country	NHS funding	Health service structure	Structure for public health workforce
England	NHS health care free at the point of access; some charges such as prescriptions, dental and optician care	Commissioning of health care through the NHS England structure; NHS providers moving to Foundation Trust status/ social enterprises	Civil service public health agency (Public Health England) for bulk of health intelligence and health protection function; some staff within NHS commissioning support or provider organisations; most health improvement staff within upper-tier local authorities (county councils and unitary authorities)
Wales	NHS health care free at the point of access; free prescriptions	NHS Health Boards – no formal purchaser– provider split	NHS public health agency covering all of Wales
Scotland	As England	NHS Health Boards – no purchaser– provider split	Health Boards
Northern Ireland	As England	NHS Health Boards – no formal purchaser– provider split	NHS public health agency covering all of Northern Ireland

Source: For detailed descriptions of each UK health system, see the UK Public Health Careers website. Available at: http://www.phorcast.org.uk/page.php?page_=1 (accessed September 2013).

Wales

The Welsh Assembly Government is responsible for the funding and oversight of the National Health Service (NHS) in Wales and other health- and social care-related bodies. As a devolved administration, Wales receives a block grant from the UK central government, which is then distributed between the different Welsh departments. Wales has three NHS regions and seven local health boards for commissioning and planning of health care through health trusts and primary care.

The public health workforce in Wales has operated on an all–Wales basis since 2003, with the formation of the National Public Health Service for Wales. Since 2010, as Public Health Wales,[259] an NHS Trust, it delivers specialist public health services to the Welsh Assembly Government, as well as support to the local health boards through Directors of Public Health (DsPH) and their teams. The Wales model contrasts with the new Public Health England (PHE) model, in place from April 2013, in that the whole of the public health workforce is employed within Public Health Wales and individual staff operate on a matrix model, balancing all–Wales responsibilities with providing local support.

Wales adopted a multidisciplinary approach to public health development from the outset of the changes for specialists in the early 2000s and, indeed, had the first non-medic to become registered on the UK Public Health Register (UKPHR) in 2003, the first defined specialist in 2006 and the first practitioner in 2011.

A key early difference in Wales was the very close links between public health and environmental health stemming from the Welsh Collaborative on the Environment during the 1990s, formed between health authority public health departments and local authority departments of environmental health. The Collaborative met regularly on an all–Wales basis to discuss a range of issues, including commissioning and housing. According to one public health consultant 'there was, therefore, a cadre of young, switched-on Environmental Health Officers (EHOs) who worked with us'.[260] This close working gave Wales a head start once Faculty of Public Health (FPH) examinations were opened to non-medics. A number of EHOs, as well as pharmacists, in Wales were among the first non-medics to sit the FPH's Part I examinations, for example.

With the opening of the UKPHR in 2003, the National Public Health Service for Wales was keen to promote an integrated public health system, employing the whole of the former health authorities' public health workforce, backed by a multidisciplinary training

---

[259] See: www.publichealthwales.wales.nhs.uk (accessed August 2013). In forming Public Health Wales, in 2009, the Wales Centre for Health was absorbed along with other all–Wales public health functions, such as screening, the Welsh Cancer Intelligence and Surveillance Unit, and the Congenital Anomalies Register and Information Service. This model contrasts with the Public Health England (PHE) model of a division between PHE functions of health protection, screening and health intelligence, and health improvement and health services public health support primarily within local government.

[260] Personal communication, 2012.

programme. It also had a policy from the early 2000s of advertised consultant in public health posts being open to suitably qualified and experienced medics and non-medics alike and to offering equal pay. As in England, there was a shortage of experienced public health medics to fill the DPH posts for the 22 health boards in Wales in 2002 and a need to recruit capacity from the non-medical workforce. 'Top-up' development support, as in England, was provided to help fill competency gaps for non-medics seeking specialist registration with the UKPHR by retrospective portfolio assessment. Development was provided and funded through the (former) Wales Centre for Health.

Wales has, therefore, been in the vanguard of multidisciplinary public health development in the UK. It participates in the national recruitment process for the higher specialist training scheme in public health, and it is piloting a process for prospective practitioner registration and advanced practitioner recognition.

Scotland

The Scottish Government Department for Health and Wellbeing is responsible for NHS Scotland, and for formulating and implementing health and community care policy. As a devolved administration, Scotland receives a block grant from the UK central government, which is then distributed between the different government departments.

NHS Scotland comprises 14 NHS Health Boards, each responsible for the planning and delivery of all health services in their own area. In addition, there are eight Special Health Boards in Scotland, which include NHS Health Scotland (Scotland's main health improvement agency) and NHS Education for Scotland (NES).

Health Boards have traditionally worked with 10 Community Health (and Care) Partnerships (CHPs). They were established on the principles of service integration, partnership-working and service redesign to ensure that patient perspectives are integrated into planning and decision-making, and that there are strong links across acute, primary and community care services. Key policy imperatives for CHPs have been shifting the balance of care to more local settings, reducing health inequalities and improving the health of local people. Following a consultation in 2012, there is a move across Scotland to replace CHPs with Health and Social Care Partnerships, which will integrate adult health and social care.

The Scottish Health Boards all have large public health departments employing consultants (mainly medical) and multidisciplinary teams delivering health improvement, health intelligence, health service and health protection services. There is a public health network spanning all Health Boards. It is likely that, in future, as in England, some NHS public health staff will become local authority employees in response to organisational change and the division of responsibilities.

Scotland has been slower to adopt multidisciplinary public health than England and Wales and has few specialist registrants on the UKPHR, as well as few consultant appointments from backgrounds other than medicine. Scottish consultants in public health medicine were more vocal in their opposition to the direction that the FPH took in the late 1990s than those in some other parts of the UK, as they wished to retain a medically led model for public health. Its higher specialist training scheme, delivered through three deaneries, has, however, been multidisciplinary since the 2013 national recruitment round. Greater Glasgow and Clyde, Lanarkshire, Ayrshire, and Arran and the Highlands Boards began to pilot the UKPHR practitioner registration programme in 2012.

On 28 May 2013, the Scottish Government published legislation (the Public Bodies (Joint Working Scotland) Bill) to integrate adult health and social care. The Highland Council had already moved the social care workforce into the NHS. There will be different options for local boards and authorities over how this will be achieved. It may well pave the way to joint posts of public health and adult social care.

Northern Ireland

The Department of Health, Social Services and Public Safety for Northern Ireland (DHSSPS) is one of 11 Northern Ireland government departments created in 1999 as part of the Northern Ireland Executive. The DHSSPS is funded from a block grant given to the Northern Ireland devolved administration from the UK Treasury. Northern Ireland ministers decide the distribution of central funds between government departments based on national priorities.

The DHSSPS carries overall responsibility to the Northern Ireland Assembly for the provision of health and social care services in Northern Ireland. Northern Ireland has had integrated health and social services since 1975. Working under the DHSSPS, the Health and Social Care Board (HSCB) is responsible for commissioning services, managing resources allocated by the DHSSPS and performance improvement.

The HSCB commissions five Health and Social Care Trusts (HSCTs) to provide health and social services across Northern Ireland. Within the HSCB, there are five Local Commissioning Groups (LCGs) responsible for the planning and resourcing of services, which cover the same geographical area as the five HSCTs.

A Northern Ireland-wide Public Health Agency (PHA) was created on 1 April 2009, integrating the three domains of public health (health improvement, health protection and health and social care quality) within a single organisation and incorporating a range of public health professionals (health promotion, health intelligence, health care, and health protection) previously employed within the HSCBs across Northern Ireland.

The PHA has responsibility for health protection, screening, health and social care research and development, safety and quality of services, and health and social well-being improvement, and provides public health, nursing and allied health professional advice to support the HSCB and its LCGs in their roles of commissioning, resource management, performance management and improvement. The PHA is organised in four divisions according to public health function and has an annual budget of around £80 million. In 2010, the PHA also assumed management of the European Centre for Connected Health (ECCH). It has close links with the HSCB and a joint commissioning plan. The Regional Director of Public Health in the PHA is also Medical Director of the HSCB. The PHA commissions alongside the board and works in tandem to deliver integrated services.

Public health in Northern Ireland is medically led and there has been almost no promotion of specialist registration of public health professionals from backgrounds other than medicine or a history of multidisciplinary public health consultant appointments. The system is marked by stability in its senior public health appointments. The training scheme has not, as yet, opened up to non-medics. Consideration is being given to setting up a pilot scheme for practitioner registration with the UKPHR. Northern Ireland has, however, a strong focus on health promotion and community development stemming from its recent turbulent history. Future organisational change will give local councils, which are reducing from 26 to 11, increased powers over well-being and thereby opportunities for public health influence.

Overall reflections

Apart from Wales, the other UK countries have not adopted multidisciplinary public health development in the same way or at the same pace as in England. It is not apparent that there was the same degree of clamour for change as there was in England during the 1990s. All four UK countries have been subject to some organisational change during the period since the late 1990s, England having seen most change and thereby most uncertainty for the public health workforce. Scotland appears to have had the most overall stability in its structure. England has recently followed Wales's and Northern Ireland's path in setting up a country-wide public health agency to encompass some of the key public health functions and services. All UK countries, moreover, have moved public health closer to local government structures. As one commentator said; 'there is much talk of the centrality of local government in public health policy and practice'.[261]

What has been achieved

- Differential adoption of the multidisciplinary movement.
- Varying opportunities for career advancement for the multidisciplinary public health workforce.
- Wales has done more to advance multidisciplinary public health practice than any other UK country and has been an early adopter of all the principal changes.

Key learning points

- Implementation of key workforce changes is dependent upon local circumstances and policies, combined with a push from the local workforces.
- Varying pace of change; cannot be imposed.

---

[261] Personal communication, 2013.

TEN

Conclusion

Introduction

Internationally, the model for the public health workforce developed in England since the late 1990s (and adopted wholly or partially by the rest of the UK countries) is unusual, both in categorising the workforce (into specialists, practitioners and the wider workforce) and in taking a holistic approach through shared (non-clinical) competency across medical and non-medically qualified public health professionals.

The approach was introduced in a piecemeal fashion rather than being undertaken strategically across the whole of the workforce from the outset.[262] Change focused initially on specialists, moving onto consideration of practitioners and then the so-called 'wider workforce'. It is only latterly that policymakers are beginning to look at the requirements, and the need, for development and underpinning competency and regulatory professional structures and frameworks for the whole of the public health workforce.

There has been more or less agreement across the whole of the UK on what is needed, at a population level, to deliver health gains and respond to health challenges. This is a competent (professional) workforce at specialist and practitioner levels, using a combination of public health technical knowledge plus skills in communication, leadership, project management and partnership-working, complemented by a 'wider workforce' geared to promote lifestyle behaviour change at an individual level, and also to influence broader aspects of public policy that impact upon health.

> **This final chapter:**
>
> - summarises what has been achieved – as well as what has not been achieved – since the 1990s to develop the public health workforce in England;
> - sets the changes in an overall context by explaining why and how they happened;

---

[262] The Witness Seminar held in 2005 (Evans and Knight, 2006) was aptly entitled *'There was no plan!'*.

- provides commentary from a range of public health professionals involved in the changes on the impact on health from the English model; and
- concludes with a reflection on the potential next stages for public health development.

What has been achieved since the 1990s to develop the public health workforce and what has been its impact on health?

According to one former President of the Faculty of Public Health (FPH):[263]

> we achieved what we set out to do – get formal recognition of multidisciplinary public health professionals as well as providing public protection.... I think it is very sustainable now – I don't think we will see a rolling back.... Has the debate now shifted to practitioners now that specialists have been more or less 'sorted'?

Pressure for change came from a perceived feeling of inequality and inequity between doctors in public health and non-medical public health – a glass ceiling in terms of career prospects and development for those from backgrounds other than medicine and a desire for equality of opportunities.

Since the late 1990s, there has been a focused attempt to build expert public health capacity in the face of increasing public health challenges and in response to changing government policies. However, according to Hunter (in a lecture at the Chartered Institute of Environmental Health on 3 September 2013[264]), national messages were mixed. The New Labour government from 1997 may have celebrated public health and permitted, for the first time, open discussion of how to tackle health inequalities, and actively acknowledged and promoted wider public health and local government's role in it, but it nevertheless introduced the *NHS plan* (DH, 2000), which sidetracked health service energies in the 2000s away from a health improvement agenda.

Most people we spoke to in preparing this book consider that a key achievement has been the creation of a substantial group of several hundred competent and accredited non-medical specialists in England

---

[263] Personal communication, 2013.
[264] Personal archive of the authors.

(and Wales) with recognised skills, most of them working in the service sector. This is a key change from the 1980s and early 1990s, when pressure for recognition came principally from distinguished academics in public health from backgrounds other than medicine.

As one interviewee stated:

> In the past only doctors could be Directors of Public Health. Now, background is irrelevant across most of the UK. But we have enabled a whole cohort to take up positions as directors, consultants, advanced practitioner leads of programmes. In the past the Faculty/Deaneries only trained doctors. Now more trainees are from backgrounds other than medicine. There is greater recognition of the team of skills needed to deliver public health – information and intelligence, health improvement. Multidisciplinary public health is sufficiently embedded and the contribution that it makes is overall accepted – a paradigm shift. Having a shared competency framework which is part of the culture has helped. There was agreement on what was core public health.[265]

Another considered that in addition to their now being a better representation of the reality of public health practice, career opportunities had been provided for people with a wide range of skills, which they could now put to the good of public health.[266]

What was achieved was not only a new personal credibility for many non-medical public health professionals, but also credibility for the whole of public health from the wider skills base on offer – as one interviewee put it: 'the public health workforce has become a broader church during the past 25 years'.[267] There has also been a recognition of the contribution to the delivery of the public health function made by public health professionals coming from a range of backgrounds, including medicine, all trained against the same competency framework. Public health in England is no longer the exclusive province of clinical public health.

Presenting hard evidence on the impact on health outcomes from this new cadre of specialists, particularly in response to shifting public health challenges, is not possible. We did receive the following two perspectives, however.

---

[265] Personal communication, 2012.
[266] Personal communication, 2012.
[267] Personal communication, 2013.

The impact of having a multidisciplinary public health workforce is a 'no-brainer':

> ensuring we have a higher proportion of our posts filled with good people than would have been the case if we just had a medical workforce. Common sense really. With a medical workforce you are limited to the number and proportion of medical graduates who want to go into public health which will always be quite small. Also bringing in people with other backgrounds means new skills.[268]

Another interviewee felt intuitively that the more complementary skills and backgrounds are brought to bear on complex problems in an organised endeavour, the more likely something will be to work: 'Health behaviour change skills, counselling skills at strategic and practitioner levels have, for example, had an outcome on smoking cessation and reductions in teenage pregnancies – we are moving right direction'.[269]

Multidisciplinary public health has also brought an important cultural contribution to public health competency. There is now more emphasis on management competency, including project management, partnership-working and team-building, that is, leadership to accompany technical competency in delivering strategic change. These skills have been particularly important in response to government policy pressure for more joint working across organisations, which marked the years from 2000.

Following a long build-up, the actual changes were also achieved in a relatively short period of time – the infrastructure, processes and funded development of specialists, to enable them to reach equivalence with medical public health, were put in place within two years. It did require a level of agreement across stakeholder organisations over what needed to happen and how. The development of a common approach to the training of public health specialists took longer.

The changes were not without risk, however, as one interviewee stated:

> there was a danger they could slip back as they had done in the 1970s when people were not properly qualified, when Medical Officers of Health roles with health protection,

---

[268] Personal communication, 2013.
[269] Personal communication, 2013.

NHS academics, health service, medical managers came together into the new specialty of community medicine. There were people who were trained to do some of public health practice but not all of it. Having got those generalist trained cohorts in the period 1980–2000 there was a danger it would slip back again with not all non-medics being competent in all the public health standards. We positioned it [the registration and regulatory processes] well to uphold standards of professional public health practice.[270]

The fears of those who considered that having a multidisciplinary public health specialist workforce would make public health less attractive as a career to doctors seem to have been largely unfounded to date. The training scheme is moving to a more or less even split between medical and non-medical recruits each year. This will need watching. As one interviewee commented:[271]

we are now in a very difficult position over the training scheme because we have run-through[272] for medical training so you have very junior people turning up competing for places on a training programme against very senior (non-medical) people and we run the risk of no longer having a multidisciplinary training programme because the one discipline we are missing is medics. Is there room for saying we need a quota of medics; we need the best medics we can get?

A real concern has been the potential lack of exposure to public health during the two years post-qualification before junior doctors have to decide which specialty they wish to enter. In the past, most doctors who ended up in public health did so after having been part-way through – or having completed – training in another specialty. When looking at cohorts of medical graduates between 1974 and 2008, Goldacre et al (2011) found that their choice of public health was typically not made until their fifth year post-graduation. This issue of flexibility within training for junior doctors across all specialties and the need to make it easier for doctors to change specialties was raised in the recent

---

[270] Personal communication, 2013.
[271] Personal communication, 2013.
[272] Junior doctors apply for their chosen specialty two years after completion of their medical degrees. For public health, then, this is five years of continuous training or four years for those who already have a Masters in Public Health.

Shape of Training review (Greenaway, 2013) and we wait to see how it might be translated into practice. Other concerns are that, because of reorganisation, young doctors may be unclear as to what kind of careers they would be entering in public health. Hunter (at lecture at the Chartered Institute of Environmental Health on 3 September 2013[273]) also referred to medical concerns of a 'dumming down' of the specialty.

Some progress was made to look at competency and development of the practitioner and wider workforces. The 2001 definitions of the public health workforce in *The report of the Chief Medical Officer's project to strengthen the public health function in England* (Donaldson, 2001) were helpful in providing a way of identifying the public health workforce, and the creation of the public health competency framework in 2008 was the first attempt to map competency across the whole workforce. There is the opportunity for recognition on a voluntary basis in certain parts of the UK for unregulated practitioners, and some local areas have strategically set up initiatives to develop public health awareness among front-line health service and local government workforces.

What has not yet been achieved?

Equivalence has been achieved for those specialists competent across all the core and defined area competencies in public health. The glass ceiling for non-medics has been removed for the higher specialist training scheme and *most* consultant in public health and Director of Public Health (DPH) appointments.[274] There has been some concern that there has been too much focus on gaining equivalence within a medical training model and that this may not be the best model for the future, particularly given the new structures for public health, where more flexibility in approach may be needed, a feeling that all that has been achieved is to create 'doctor clones'. Equally, as has been outlined in previous chapters, the medical–non-medical tensions have not gone away, emerging at each reorganisation.

Regulation is currently still voluntary for non-medical specialists, although, since 2003, NHS consultant in public health appointments have required regulation by the UK Public Health Register (UKPHR) in the case of non-medical applicants, apart from dental public health (regulated by the General Dental Council). The status of those registered as defined specialists with the UKPHR in the long term is not clear

---

[273] Personal archive of the authors.

[274] Some posts with clinical content remain open to those with a medical qualification only, such as the Chief Medical Officer and other very senior posts.

– for example, whether they will be included within the proposed statutory regulation of non-medical (generalist) specialists and whether there will be prospective training or development routes.

Once new non-medical DPH appointment processes were in place, there was a strategic approach taken to the rapid development of non-medical specialists by the Department of Health (DH) and national public health organisations to ensure public protection. This has not happened for practitioners even though they have been more or less identifiable in the workplace since 2006. Formal practitioner registration and regulation is still partial – some being statutory, some voluntary – and, indeed, there is, as yet, no consistent view over whether it is needed or not for the whole practitioner workforce.

There is no clear pathway for advancement or recognition at different career points for practitioners, particularly at advanced practitioner level. Career paths remain idiosyncratic. Public Health England (PHE) is likely to focus on its own non-medical clinical scientists and health intelligence practitioner staff in the first instance. The lack of clear career pathways and development for the practitioner workforce has led to relatively junior members of staff considering application for defined specialist status and, likewise, more senior members of staff considering UKPHR practitioner registration – simply because there appear to them to be no other options for formal recognition.

One interviewee for the book felt, on reflection, that it would have been strategically better to have started with practitioners and worked up to specialists, although she recognised that this was not possible given the pressure in 2002 to provide public protection for non-medical DPH appointments.[275] There is concern that by achieving specialist recognition without accompanying structures for practitioners, we have merely raised expectations unrealistically.

We still cannot count the workforce, a problem that will become more acute in a workforce no longer primarily employed within the health service, but dispersed across a whole range of different organisations. There is also no longer cohesion across public health organisations. As one interviewee commented, 'we still have a Faculty which is very exclusive'; and another, 'we're faced with massive changes and we're not talking together and facing the same direction'.[276]

Boosting academic public health capacity remains a long-term problem and there are particular inequities between medical and

[275] Personal communication, 2013.
[276] Personal communication, 2012, 2013.

non-medical public health researchers in terms of opportunities for advancement and salaries.

Public health leadership, including developing new generations of leaders, remains an issue within the public health workforce. With the 2002 health service changes, many senior public health leaders, for example, some Health Authority DsPH, chose to leave the service rather than work in much smaller Primary Care Trusts (PCTs) with lower status. This was at a time when 99 Health Authority posts were replaced with 303 PCTs. Although non-medical public health specialists boosted senior-level capacity from 2003, having sufficient professionals of the right calibre, particularly as roles become ever-more complex at each reorganisation, remains a challenge. In the system from April 2013, there are 152 upper-tier councils with DPH positions, as well as 15 PHE Centres.

Many of these issues were recognised in the *Public health workforce strategy* (DH et al, 2013) for England and outlined in the comments during the consultation on the draft. The pace of change and development had slowed, however, from 2008, particularly during the transition from 2010 to implementation of the new structures in April 2013. There is still, at times, an uneasy relationship in public health between doctors and those not medically trained, the dormant tensions having been reawakened during the transition. There are new tensions between public health and adult social care in some local authorities. It will take time to gain new momentum for workforce change and development.

The context for change

The journey to development of a multidisciplinary public health workforce has been patchy, marked by periods of intense activity and periods where little progress was made. According to Hunter et al (2007, p 44), there has never been a shared philosophy governing public health, 'with the result that old and new models of public health compete with each other, resurface from time to time, and jostle for position and supremacy instead of co-existing in a balanced approach'.

Most of the public health workforce in England from 1974 to 2013 has worked from a health service base (with the exception of staff within the Health Protection Agency [HPA] from 2002). This has brought both advantages and disadvantages. Advantages stem from the prominent positions within senior management structures in the health service afforded to public health professionals, providing opportunities to influence health strategies, planning and commissioning of health care;

disadvantages from the continual subjection to organisational change with each incoming government or policy change. One interviewee commented that his proudest achievement was to preserve local and regional public health posts for as long as possible – while there were opposing attempts to remove them at every reorganisation, particularly from the local layer – thereby ensuring that there was always a senior public health role in the most local population unit.

Since 1974, there has been no settled employment structure for the public health workforce in England. Because most worked within the management and administrative tiers of the health service (until the creation of the HPA in 2002), the public health workforce, along with managerial colleagues, have had to go through organisational change, seemingly occurring at ever-shorter intervals. Constant reorganisation of the health and public health system in England has tended to stem from a prevailing view that each previous system was dysfunctional, had too many weak links and did not meet the prevailing ideology of the government at the time. Although each reorganisation has provided a new set of opportunities for the public health workforce, a weariness with change may have prevented them being seized in time before the next reorganisation took place. There is less stability and 'protection'. One interviewee compared the situation post-1974, when the bulk of public health moved from local government to the NHS, with the previous relatively stable position from 1948, when Medical Officers of Health could provide professional opinions without risk to their positions and were not subject to constant reorganisation.[277]

Constant organisational change also hampers implementation of major workforce planning and development, which can take years to fully work through. The public health workforce changes in the late 1990s and early 2000s appeared to be helped by a willingness of successive generations of stakeholder leads to maintain the momentum for change. The role of the DH was crucial as an early sponsor of change and a funder of development, and in using its influence to make things happen. This is in marked contrast to subsequent divisions from 2008, particularly the failure of national public health organisations to present a united front.

It is not clear how instrumental the relatively weak position of clinical public health that existed in the 1980s and 1990s was in enabling the creation of a multidisciplinary specialist public health workforce. Their relatively new provenance in any significant numbers within the health service from 1974 and the time it took to gain credibility and status

---

[277] Personal communication, 2013.

with medical consultant colleagues meant that some public health doctors have consistently taken a defensive stance in the face of potential competition from non-medical public health colleagues. Certainly, anxieties about status and salary differentials between the medical and non-medical public health workforce have tended to emerge at each health service reorganisation. One interviewee commented on the 'growing lip service to the cause [among public health doctors] as it became politically correct to be seen to support a multidisciplinary public health workforce – contrasted with those who were sincerely in favour of it'.[278]

The English model in an international context

Much of the contemporary focus on public health workforce development around the world appears to have its origins in the perceived need by governments to ensure sufficient capacity to protect against major and unexpected threats to population health, such as pandemic disease or terrorism. The necessary capacity is usually described in terms of competencies required to respond to such threats to public health rather than the core discipline or occupational background of those employed to deliver public health functions. Indeed, during the past decade, there have been projects to identify and articulate public health competencies in many places, including the US, Australia and the European Union.

A clear policy description was articulated in the US Centers for Disease Control and Prevention (CDC)'s *Public health surveillance workforce of the future* (Drehobl et al, 2012):

> Although the astute clinician remains a crucial link in surveillance, persons from other disciplines are often the first to recognize events that require prompt interventions of public health workers ... workforce initiatives are needed to ensure that the right talent is in the right job at the right time. Such efforts would focus on enhancing the skills and availability of public health workers and also the diverse disciplines.

Alongside the recognition that the public health workforce must be diverse is a somewhat uncomfortable recognition that there is little evidence that the composition of the workforce is correlated with

---

[278] Personal communication, 2012.

its achievements. Beaglehole and Dal Poz (2003) point to the lack of attention in both developed and developing nations to building the public health workforce, and to the lack of evidence to support the assertion that investment in the public health workforce will influence population health, although they do suggest that it is reasonable to assume that this is the case. Gursky and Batni (2010) assert that we need a strong multidisciplinary global public health workforce – an aspiration that we would support strongly, despite the lack of research evidence to prove its efficacy.

Another factor resonating from international experience is the newly rediscovered focus on public health education for doctors and aspiring doctors. There have been initiatives by some medical schools in this country and others to raise the profile of public health content of undergraduate education – for example, the Harvard (Finkelstein et al, 2008) initiative that comprised new content in the first-year pre-clinical course, the aim being to equip future doctors to contribute to the response to public health emergencies, but not necessarily to develop future cohorts of public health specialists.

An area where the UK remains different from many other countries is the ongoing tension and strict separation in some countries between public health and health care delivery. As a result, there have been initiatives to integrate public health and health care delivery, and, in particular, public health and primary care. Until the recent NHS reforms in England, public health was integral to the health care system, but with the separation of local public health teams from the NHS, the situation may now change and the need for such initiatives may emerge in England, too. So, while in England, the 'integration' agenda is currently about integrating health and social care, we need to be aware that potential opportunities for highly effective, integrated public health and health and social care systems could be missed.

Finally, in this brief summary of the international context, we are reminded that terminology is constantly evolving. Galindo et al (2010) point out that 'even Linguistics has directed its efforts to define diverse terms that denote cross-border information exchange', and describe what they call the semantic shift from multi-, to inter-, to cross-, to trans-disciplinary activity to reflect the tasks of modern societies. So, while we have addressed the evolution of the multidisciplinary public health workforce, on the global stage, we perhaps need to consider deploying some of these newer terms to describe the ever-evolving public health workforce.

Time for a new paradigm?

The English model for the public health professional workforce since 1974 has been built on the medical structure of a hierarchical pyramid, with the consultant at the top and others in training/support roles. Broadening the top of the pyramid with the addition of consultants and specialists from backgrounds other than medicine has not changed this structure. What is different about public health is that those in 'support' roles are not all necessarily clearly defined, in specific training or in a recognised grading, each with its own qualifications and status. This structure prompted the initial move for multidisciplinary recognition at specialist level and the pressure now for recognition at different levels for practitioners.

We will need a new paradigm for the future public health workforce given the fragmentation following the implementation of the Coalition government's reforms. When the bulk of the workforce was employed within either local government (before 1974) or the NHS (1974–2013), it was possible to have some consistency in approach to titles, appointments, profiles, terms and conditions. Now, with a workforce split across a myriad of different employers, this is no longer possible. Further, in many organisations, there may be lone public health professionals.

The pattern now is for constant organisational change and restructuring. To fit with this and still deliver public health outcomes, we need a professional public health workforce, confident in its skills and knowledge and flexible enough to cope with different challenges and different partners, as well as different employer organisations. Therefore, a model is required that does not rely on a single employer, specific titles or gradings, but which is based around a recognised skill set and competencies, continuing professional development, and accreditation or regulation at appropriate points, whether statutory or voluntary. Having a professionally agreed competency framework that spans the whole public health workforce (periodically updated to reflect new public health challenges and new evidence concerning effective response) – a 'passport for public health' recognised by employers across all sectors and professional 'homes' for the workforce to provide support (in the way that the FPH does for public health professionals at specialist level) – may provide the best way forward for a dispersed workforce model.

And what of the future for the English public health workforce?

The acknowledged combination of skills required to deliver public health services across the three domains of public health practice (health protection, health improvement and health and social care services) has remained remarkably stable over time, with different elements coming to the fore over the years in response to shifting public health issues and challenges that need to be addressed. It is a story since 1974 of constant adaptation to new circumstances. A key change since the early 1970s, however, is the increasing recognition that these issues cannot be addressed, or the challenge response led, solely by those from medical backgrounds. A more eclectic base for skills and range of approaches adapted for different settings and functions, as well as an increased and competent workforce, will be needed if a real difference is to be made to health outcomes. We need to embrace new players, such as those within local government – social workers, teachers, engineers, housing officers and planners. Where we are now on the journey, therefore, is part-way through developing a coherent multidisciplinary public health and well-being workforce at all levels and comprising a range of different backgrounds.

There are new major national organisational players on the public health scene from 2013. This will, inevitably, have an impact on the public health workforce in England and how it develops in the next few years – specifically, local government, with its additional public health responsibilities, and PHE, who are now the two main employers of the public health workforce.

It remains to be seen how PHE will interface with the other national and local public health organisations and what role it will, in time, play in influencing public health policy and the development and evolution of the public health workforce. What is clear, however, is that the public health workforce in England, unlike the other UK countries, is now, to a large extent, fragmented and divided across different cultures – civil service, local government and, to a much lesser extent, the health service. What the impact of this will be is unclear. The current FPH President has a vision for the future of the public health workforce of a Royal College that embraces all those in public health or with an interest in public health, linked by a common generic basic training and having numerous 'faculties' representing different special interests. Interestingly, to date, there has been only one non-medic voted into any of the senior FPH officer positions (in 2014); indeed, few have stood for election. It is not clear why this should be the case.

There seems to be general agreement that enhancing local government's capacity and capability to influence the social determinants of health will bring the potential for substantial benefits in health outcomes. Local government could see the resurgence of health promotion and community development in a way that has not been seen since the 1980s. Hunter (at a lecture at the Chartered Institute of Environmental Health on 3 September 2013[279]), in looking at the possibilities for the future, referred to public health as being 'unchained' from where it has been (embedded within the NHS), possibly becoming 'unshackled from its biomedical model' and able to fully embrace the social model of health determinants. This will require new skills and competencies, particularly in influencing others engaged in health improvement and well-being, as well as new approaches to presenting evidence and knowledge exchange – a focus on 'softer', relational, rather than technical, skills. Developing these skills in DsPH and their senior teams is pressing if they are to be able to operate effectively in a different cultural and political context. He also considered that, in local government at least, the former paradigm of dividing the public health workforce across specialists, practitioners and the wider workforce may well need to change.

Moving away from a biomedical model also means public health moving away from the health service. Despite various governments' stated policy for the health service to begin to focus on health and prevention, as well as health care, in reality, agendas since the late 1970s have tended to principally address issues of quality of health care delivery. There is a risk of further loss of valuable influence from public health by this latest reorganisation. Have the 2013 reforms swung too far in the 'wrong' direction? Public health has always remained strongest when it can influence across all sectors.

There are some fears, however, of what the move to local government will mean for the health improvement workforce in particular – whether it will cope with local democratic structures effectively, and whether it will be subject to reductions in the current economic climate or downgrading once the ring-fenced funding ends.

In the longer term, it is less clear whether local government will be the 'home' for the multidisciplinary public health workforce working in health improvement, and whether medical public health will work primarily in PHE alongside health intelligence and health protection colleagues. As one interviewee commented:

---

[279] Personal archive of the authors.

there is a real danger that you end up with the medics going into PHE and PHE becoming a silo which is irrelevant to local government and then public health loses the weight of its argument. The only way this will work is if local authorities themselves become public health organisations. If you have all the medics with all their power base moving into PHE then you've fractured public health and moved back to the 1970s.[280]

Provided that the recommended underpinning infrastructure of a skills passport and public health competency framework is implemented, England's *Public health workforce strategy* (DH et al, 2013) should go some way in providing a framework for development of the practitioner public health workforce. A number of strategic issues relating to formal professional recognition and career development remain unresolved, however.

Because the English system is now so far removed from the models adopted for public health across the rest of the UK, it is not clear what the impact of what happens in England in the future will be on the rest of the UK. The *Public health workforce strategy* applies to England but some of the content will have potential implications across the other UK countries, such as development of a skills passport for public health and statutory regulation of non-medical public health specialists. The possibility of Scottish independence simply adds to the uncertainty of UK-wide workforce development.

The strategy did not address the public health role and development of the wider, front-line workforce, but it is likely that this will be of considerable interest to the new health education structures – Health Education England (HEE) and its Local Education and Training Boards – as they strive to improve health and save money. HEE has the UK public health competency framework within its public health careers website, and is, therefore, well placed to deliver the 'Making every contact count' (MECC) initiative.[281]

Has the time come, too, to revive the public health and primary care agenda with the new GP-led Clinical Commissioning Groups driving secondary care commissioning and attempts once more to shift services from acute to community care? A number of deaneries are already setting up public health placements or teaching in population health as part of formal GP training.

[280] Personal communication, 2011.
[281] As outlined by the Future Forum report of 2012 during the period of transition to the new health system in England from April 2013 (Field, 2012).

Despite the constant reorganisation and change that the workforce is subject to, there does not appear, at present, to be any lack of interest in recruits. Junior doctor medical interest, despite fears, remains strong and there is intense competition from applicants from a range of backgrounds for the annual recruitment round into the formal higher specialist training scheme leading to entry into the consultant and specialist-level workforce. There is no lessening of popularity of those wishing to undertake Masters in Public Health courses and then move into public health roles, or, for existing practitioners, to apply for voluntary practitioner regulation where schemes exist.

The public health workforce in England has come a long way since the 1970s. We understand better who is in the workforce, we are clear on its role and contribution to public health outcomes, and we know the competencies needed at different levels within the workforce. The future challenge is to continue to recognise, harness, refine and develop these skills in a holistic way to maximise the multidisciplinary contribution while remaining fleet of foot and resilient enough to ensure that the workforce can adapt to what seems to be inevitable future service reconfiguration.

References

Acheson, D. (1988) *Public health in England: the report of the Committee of Inquiry into the Future Development of the Public Health Function*, Cm 289, London: HMSO.

Acheson, D. (1998) *Independent inquiry into health inequalities*, London: Stationery Office.

Ashton, J. (1999) 'Past and present public health in Liverpool', in S. Griffiths and D. Hunter (eds) *Perspectives in public health*, Oxford: Radcliffe Medical Press, pp 23–33.

Ashton, J. and Seymour, H. (1988) *The new public health: the Liverpool experience*, Milton Keynes: Open University Press.

ASPH (Association of School of Public Health) (2008) 'Confronting the public health workforce crisis: ASPH statement on the public health workforce', February. Available at: http://www.asph.org/UserFiles/PHWFShortage0208.pdf (accessed March 2014).

Ball, L. and Nasr, N. (2011) 'A qualitative exploration of a health trainer programme in two UK Primary Care Trusts', *Perspectives in Public Health*, vol 131, no 1, pp 24-31.

Bartley, M. (1992) *Authorities and partisans*, Edinburgh: Edinburgh University Press.

Beaglehole, R. and Dal Poz, M.R. (2003) 'Public health workforce: challenges and policy issues', *Human Resources for Health*, vol 1, no 4, pp 1–4.

Berridge, V. (2007) 'Multidisciplinary public health: what sort of victory?', *Public Health*, vol 121, pp 404–8.

Berridge, V., Christie, D.A. and Tansey, E.M. (2006) *Public health in the 1980s and 1990s: decline and rise?*, transcript of a witness seminar held by the Wellcome Trust Centre for the History of Medicine at UCL, London, 12 October 2004 (referred to as Witness Seminar 1 in the footnotes).

Bimpe, O., Killoran, A. and Rae, M. (2006) 'Health trainers: a new public health practitioner in England', *Ph.com, The newsletter of the Faculty of Public Health*, FPH, London, June.

BMA (British Medical Association) Parliamentary Unit (2011) *Maintaining the specialist public health workforce* (Personal archive of the authors).

Brown, J.S. and Learmonth, A. (2005) 'Mind the gap: developing the PH workforce in the North East and Yorkshire and Humber Regions: a scoping stakeholder study', *Public Health*, vol 119, pp 32–8.

Brown, R.G.S. (1970) *Reorganising the National Health Service*, Oxford: Blackwell.

Brown, S., Burns, D., Chapel, H., Cronin, D., Evans, D., Gray, S., Howard, J., Kendall, L., Lewendon, G., Mackenzie, I., Miles, D., Morgan, K. and Orme, J. (2007) 'Public health leadership in the real world: the role of the DPH', *Public Health Medicine*, vol 6, no 2, pp 58–60.

Burke, S., Meyrick, J. and Speller, V. (2001) *The public health skills audit research report*, London: Health Development Agency.

Calman, K. (1998) *Chief Medical Officer's project to strengthen the public health function in England – report of emerging findings*, London: Department of Health.

Carlson, C. (2008) 'Experiences with using the public health skills and career framework', *Ph.com, The newsletter of the Faculty of Public Health*, FPH, London, December, p 11.

Cochrane, A.L. (1972) *Effectiveness and efficiency: random reflections on health services*, The Nuffield Provincial Hospitals Trust.

Cooper, R. (2005) 'Modernising public health careers', *Ph.com, The newsletter of the Faculty of Public Health*, FPH, London, March, pp 10-11.

Cornish, Y. and Knight, T. (2000) *Exploring public health career paths: an overview of career opportunities in public health and health improvement in England*, Birmingham: South East Institute of Public Health, The University of Birmingham.

Cornish, Y. and Knight, T. (2002) *Specialists in public health – proceeding to part II FPHM membership*, Tunbridge Wells: Centre for Health Services Studies, University of Kent and Health Service Management Centre.

Cosford, P., O'Mahony, M., Angell, E., Bickler, G., Crawshaw, S., Glencross, J., Horsley, S.S., McCloskey, B., Puleston, R., Seare, N. and Tobin, M.D. (2006) 'Public health professionals' perceptions towards provision of health protection in England: a survey of expectations of PCTs and Health Protection Units in the delivery of health protection', *BMC Public Health*, vol 6, no 297, pp 1–11.

Court Report (1976) *Fit for the future: The report of the Committee on Child Health Services*, (chairman S.D.M. Court), Cm 6684, London: HMSO.

Crown, J. (1999) 'The practice of public health medicine', in S. Griffiths and D.J. Hunter (eds) *Perspectives in public health*, Oxford: Radcliffe Publishing Ltd, p 219.

Dawson, S., Sherval, J., Mole, J. and Mole, V. (1996) 'In or out of management? Dilemma and developments in public health medicine in England', in J. Leopold, I. Glover and M. Hughes (eds) *Beyond reason? The National Health Service and the limitations of management*, London: Avebury, pp 157–72.

DH (Department of Health) (1989) *Working for patients: the health service caring for the 1990s*, Cm 555, London: HMSO.

DH (1992) *Health of the nation: a strategy for health in England*, Cm 1986, London: HMSO.

DH (1993) *Public health: responsibilities of the NHS and roles of others*, Advice of the committee set up to undertake a review of HC(88)64 (Abrams Committee) (HSG(93)56), London.

DH (1998) *Our healthier nation: a contract for health*, Cm 3852, 1 January, London: Stationery Office.

DH (1999a) *Saving lives: our healthier nation*, Cm 4386, London: Stationery Office.

DH (1999b) *Reducing health inequalities: an action report*, 1 January, London: Stationery Office.

DH (2000) *NHS plan: a plan for investment: a plan for reform*, Cm 4818-1, 1 July, London: Stationery Office.

DH (2001) *Shifting the balance of power within the NHS: securing delivery*, July, London.

DH (2002a) *Shifting the balance of power: the next steps*, 4 January, London.

DH (2002b) *Getting ahead of the curve: a strategy for combating infectious diseases including other aspects of health protection*, 10 January, London.

DH (2004a) *Modernising medical careers: the next steps*, 15 April, London.

DH (2004b) *Choosing health: making healthier choices easier*, Cm 6374, 16 November, London: Stationery Office.

DH (2004c) *Agenda for Change: final agreement*, 22 December, London.

DH (2005) *Commissioning a patient led NHS, letter from Sir Nigel Crisp, CEO of the NHS to NHS CEOs*, 28 July, London.

DH (2006) *The NHS in England: the operating framework for 2007/8*, December, London.

DH (2007) *World class commissioning – vision, competencies, assessment framework, support and development framework*, December, London.

DH (2010a) *Equity and excellence: liberating the NHS*, Cm 7881, 12 July, London: Stationery Office.

DH (2010b) *Healthy lives, healthy people: our strategy for public health in England*, 30 November, London.

DH (2010c) *Review of the regulation of public health professionals*, Gabriel Scally, Regional Director of Public Health for the South West, 30 November, London.

DH (2010d) *NHS outcomes framework*, 20 December, London.

DH (2010e) *Modernising scientific careers: the UK way forward*, 26 February, London.

DH (2011) *Health Visitor implementation plan 2011–15: a call to action*, February, London.

DH (2012a) *Public health outcomes framework*, 23 January, London.

DH (2012b) *Healthy lives, healthy people: towards a workforce strategy for the public health system – consultation document*, 27 March, London.

DH (2013) *Healthy lives, healthy people: towards a workforce strategy for the public health system: a consultation. Summary of responses*, 3 May, London.

DH, Public Health England and Local Government Association (2013) *Healthy lives, healthy people: a public health workforce strategy*, 3 May.

DHSS (Department of Health and Social Security) (1972a) *National Health Service reorganisation: England. Consultative document*, Cm 5055, London: HMSO.

DHSS (1972b) *The working party on medical administrators* (Hunter Report), London: HMSO.

DHSS (1980) *Inequalities in health: the Black Report*, London: HMSO.

DHSS (1983) *NHS management inquiry report* (Griffiths Report), London.

DHSS (1986) *Report of the Committee of Inquiry into an outbreak of food poisoning at Stanley Royd Hospital*, Cm 9716, London: HMSO.

Donaldson, L. (2001) *The report of the Chief Medical Officer's project to strengthen the public health function in England*, London: Department of Health.

Donaldson, L. (2002) *Unfinished business: proposals for reform of the senior house officer grade. A paper for consultation*, August, DH.

Drehobl, P.A., Roush, S.W., Stover, B.H. and Koo, D. (2012) 'Public health surveillance workforce of the future', *Morbidity and Mortality Weekly Report (MMWR)*, Centers for Disease Control and Prevention, vol 61, no 3, pp 25-9.

Dunkley, R. and Wright, J. (2010) 'Academic public health: summary of emerging findings from a review of the workforce perspective of academic public health in England', Solutions for Public Health, unpublished report for the Department of Health, September.

Evans, D. and Adams, L. (2007) 'Through the glass ceiling – and back again: the experience of two of the first non-medical Directors of Public Health in England', *Public Health*, vol 121, no 6, pp 426–31.

Evans, D. and Dowling, S. (2002) 'Developing a multi-disciplinary public health specialist workforce: training implications of current UK policy', *Journal of Epidemiology and Community Health*, vol 56, pp 744–7.

Evans, D. and Knight, T. (eds) (2006) *'There was no plan!' – the origins and development of multidisciplinary public health in the UK: report of the witness seminar held at the University of the West of England on Monday 7 November 2005*, Bristol: University of the West of England, Faculty of Health and Social Care (referred to as Witness Seminar 2 in the footnotes).

Field, S. (chair) (2012) *NHS Future Forum summary report – second phase*, January, London.

Finkelstein, J.A., McMahon, G.T., Peters, A., Cadigan, R., Biddinger, P. and Simon S.R. (2008) 'Teaching population health as a basic science at Harvard Medical School', *Academic Medicine*, vol 83, no 4, pp 332-7.

FPH (Faculty of Public Health) of the Royal Colleges of Physicians of the United Kingdom (2004) *Annual report of the board*, London: Faculty of Public Health.

FPH of the Royal Colleges of Physicians of the United Kingdom (2005) *Annual report*, London: Faculty of Public Health.

FPH of the Royal Colleges of Physicians of the United Kingdom (2006) *Annual review*, London: Faculty of Public Health.

FPHM (Faculty of Public Health Medicine) of the Royal Colleges of Physicians of the United Kingdom (2001) *Annual report of the board*, London: Faculty of Public Health Medicine.

FPHM of the Royal Colleges of Physicians of the United Kingdom (2002) *Annual report of the board*, London: Faculty of Public Health Medicine.

Galindo, F., Guidotti, M., Gulevich, V., Gursky, E. and Kolesnikov, S. (2010) 'Information sharing in knowledge society', in A. Trufanov, A. Rossodivita, M. Guidotti (eds) *Pandemics and bioterrorism*, IOS Press.

Goldacre, M.J., Laxton, L., Lambert, T.W. and Webster, P. (2011) 'Career choices for public health: cohort studies of graduates from UK medical schools', *Journal of Public Health*, vol 33, no 4, pp 616–23.

Gray, S. and Sandberg, E. (2006) *The specialist public health workforce in the UK 2005 survey: a report for the board of the Faculty of Public Health*, London: Faculty of Public Health.

Gray, S. and Sandberg, E. (2008) *Specialist public health workforce in the UK: a report for the Board of the Faculty of Public Health*, London: Faculty of Public Health.

Green, S. (2007) 'Health trainers – making a difference', *Ph.com, The newsletter of the Faculty of Public Health*, London: FPH, December, p 13.

Greenaway, D. (2013) *Securing the future of excellent patient care: final report of the independent review*, Shape of Training, October, www.shapeoftraining.co.uk (accessed February 2014).

Griffiths, J. and Dark, P. (2005) *Shaping the future of public health: promoting health in the NHS*, Department of Health, July.

Griffiths, J. and Sugarman, R. (2004) *Scoping study, UK public health register* (unpublished).

Griffiths, S., Thorpe, A. and Wright, J. (2005) *Change and development in specialist public health practice*, Oxford: Radcliffe Publishing.

Griffiths, S., Crown, J. and McEwen, J. (2007) 'The role of the Faculty of Public Health (Medicine) in developing a multidisciplinary public health profession in the UK', *Public Health*, vol 121, pp 420–5.

Gursky, E.A. and Batni, S.R. (2010) 'Learning from catastrophe – lessons for pandemic planning', in A. Trufanov et al (eds) *Pandemics and bioterrorism*, IOS Press.

Hannaway, C., Plsek, P. and Hunter, D.J. (2007) 'Developing leadership and management for health', in D.J. Hunter (ed) *Managing for health*, Abingdon: Routledge, pp 148–73.

Hunt, P. (2001) 'The Future of Public Health', speech to the Faculty of Public Health Medicine, Royal College of Physicians, 13 November. Available at: http://webarchive.nationalarchives.gov.uk/+/www.dh.gov.uk/en/MediaCentre/Speeches/Speecheslist/DH_4000629 (accessed July 2011).

Hunter, D.J. (2013) Extract from unpublished chapter for *Perspectives on Public Health* series sent to authors

Hunter, D.J., Marks, L. and Smith, K. (2007) *The public health system in England: a scoping study*, Centre for Public Policy and Health, Durham University School for Health, November.

Hunter, D.J., Marks, L. and Smith, K.E. (2010) *The public health system in England*, Bristol: The Policy Press

IOM (Institute of Medicine) (1988) *The future of public health*, 1 January. Available at: www.iom.edu (accessed March 2014).

IOM (2002) *Who will keep the public healthy? Educating public health professionals for the 21st century*, November. Available at: www.iom.edu (accessed March 2014).

IOM (2007) *Training physicians for public health careers*, 6 June. Available at: www.iom.edu (accessed March 2014).

Jones, L. and Earle, S. (2009) 'Back to the future: reflections on multidisciplinary public health', in J. Douglas, S. Earle, S. Handsley, L.J. Jones, C.L. Lloyd and S. Spurr (eds) *A reader in promoting public health, challenge and controversy* (2nd edn), Sage Publications Ltd in Association with the Open University.

Klein, R. (2006) *The new politics of the NHS: from creation to reinvention* (5th edn), Abingdon: Radcliffe Publishing.

Lalonde, M. (1974) *A new perspective on the health of Canadians: a working document (the Lalonde Report)*, Ottawa: Government of Canada.

Lessof, S., Dumelow, C. and McPherson, K. (1999) *Feasibility study of the case for national standards for specialist practice in public health – a report for the NHS Executive. Cancer and Public Health Unit*, London: London School of Hygiene and Tropical Medicine.

Lewis, J. (1986) *What price community medicine? The philosophy, practice and politics of public health since 1999*, Sussex: Wheatsheaf Books.

Lewis, J. (1987) 'From public health to community medicine: the wider context', in S. Farrow (ed) *The public health challenge*, London: Hutchinson Education, pp 87–100.

Lewis, J. (1991) 'The public's health: philosophy and practice in Britain in the twentieth century', in E. Fee and R. Acheson (eds) *A history of education in public health*, Oxford: Oxford University Press, pp 195–229.

Lock, K. and Sim, F. (2009) 'Public health in the United Kingdom', in R. Beaglehole and R. Bonita (eds) *Global public health: a new era* (2nd edn), Oxford: Oxford University Press, pp 63–8.

Marmot, M. (2010) *Fair society, healthy lives. Strategic review of health inequalities in England post 2010. The Marmot Review*, February, London: University College London.

Maryon-Davis, A. (2010) 'The changing public health workforce', in F. Campbell (ed) *The social determinants of health and the role of local government*, London: Improvement and Development Agency.

McErlain, S. (1998) 'Multidisciplinary public health development: status of national and regional initiatives', unpublished briefing paper for the Regional Directors of Public Health, South West Regional Office, 16 July.

McEwen, J. (2004) 'Registered interest?', *Public Health News*, 1 March, pp 10–12.

McPherson, K. (1999) 'The fate of non-medics working in public health. Letter to the editor', *Journal of Epidemiological Community Health*, vol 53, p 128.

McPherson, K. (2001) 'For and against: public health does not need to be led by doctors. Education and debate', *British Medical Journal*, vol 322 (30 June), p 1593.

Milburn, A. (2000) *A healthier nation and a healthier economy: the contribution of a modern NHS*, speech at the London School of Economics Annual Lecture, 8 March. Available at: www.webarchive.nationalarchives.gov.uk/+/www.dh.gov.uk/en/MediaCentre/Speech/SpeechesList/DH_4000761 (accessed July 2011).

Mitchell, D. and Lassiter, S. (2006) 'Addressing healthcare disparities and increasing workforce diversity: the next step for the dental, medical and public health professions', *American Journal of Public Health*, vol 96, no 12, pp 2093–7.

Nelson, A., De Normanville, C., Payne, K. and Kelly, M. (2013) 'Making every contact count: an evaluation', *Public Health*, vol 127 (July), pp 653–60.

O'Hara, G. (2007) *From dreams to disillusionment: economic and social planning in 1960s' Britain*, Basingstoke: Palgrave Macmillan.

Orme, J., De Viaggiani, N. and Knight, T. (2007) 'Missed opportunities? Locating health promotion within multidisciplinary public health', *Public Health*, vol 121, no 6, pp 414–19.

Packham, C. and Robinson, M. (2011) 'Public health medicine skills in the NHS: vital and very vulnerable', *British Journal of General Practice*, vol 588, p 462.

Pilkington, P., Dowling, S., Barnes, G., Lindfield, T. and Prichard, A. (2007) 'Trainees' experiences of multidisciplinary public health training schemes in England', *Public Health*, vol 121, pp 432–7.

Pittam, G. and Wright, J. (2011) 'The role of the Director of Public Health in England', *Perspectives in Public Health*, vol 131, pp 17–18.

Porter, D. (ed) (1994) 'The history of public health and the modern state', *Rodopi*, 1 January.

Richardson, A., Duggan, M. and Hunter, D. (1994) 'Adapting to new tasks: the role of public health physicians in purchasing health care', Nuffield Institute for Health, Leeds University.

Roden, A. and Owen-Smith, A. (2008) 'A brief history of the rise and fall of the School Medical Service in England', *Public Health*, vol 122, no 3, pp 268–70.

RSPH (Royal Society for Public Health) (2014) *The views of local public health teams working in local authorities*, February. Available at: www. rsph.org.uk (accessed February 2014).

Sackett, D.L., Rosenberg, W.M., Gray, J.A., Haynes, R.B. and Richardson, W.S. (1996) 'Evidence based medicine: what it is and what it isn't', *British Medical Journal*, vol 312, no 7023, pp 71–2.

Seebohm Report (1968) *Report of the Committee on Local Authority and Allied Personal Social Services*, Cm 3703, London: HMSO.

Sim, F.M. (2007) 'Teaching Public Health Networks: connecting with "Shaping the Future"', *Journal of the Royal Society for the Promotion of Health*, vol 127, no 5, pp 227–30.

Sim, F. (2012) '2012: What health impact?', *Journal of Epidemiology and Community Health*, vol 66, pp 667–9.

Sim, F., Schiller, G. and Walters, R. (2002) *Public health workforce planning for London: mapping the public health function in London: a report to the DHSC*, London: DH Directorate of Health and Social Care.

Sim, F., Lock, K. and McKee, M. (2007) 'Maximising the contribution of the public health workforce: the English experience', *Bulletin of the WHO*, vol 85, no 12, pp 935–9.

Skills for Health (2004) *National Occupational Standards for Public Health.* Access via: http://nos.ukces.org.uk/Pages/results.aspx [search under '2004 national occupational standards for public health'].

Skills for Health (2008) 'UK public health skills and career framework', April. Access via www.phorcast.org.uk (accessed March 2014).

Smith, A., Jacobson, B. and Whitehead, M. (eds) (1991) *The nation's health: a strategy for the 1990s*, King's Fund.

Smith, D.C. and Davies, L. (1997) 'Who contributes to the public health function?', *Journal of Public Health Medicine*, vol 19, no 4, pp 451–6.

Snow, S., Kessel, A. and Buckley, E. (eds) (2013) *'Joining all the pieces together': the origins and development of the Health Protection Agency 2003–2013*, Report of the Witness Seminar held at the HPA 15 January, Public Health England, April.

Social Exclusion Unit (2001) *A new commitment to neighbourhood renewal: national strategy action plan*, Report, January, Cabinet Office.

Somervaille, L (2005) 'Welcome to the first formally trained public health specialist', *Ph.com. The newsletter of the Faculty of Public Health*, London: FPH, March, p 17.

Somervaille, L. (2008) 'Development of regulation for public health practitioners', *Ph.com, the newsletter of the Faculty of Public Health*, London: FPH, December.

Somervaille, L. and Griffiths, R. (1995) *The training and career development needs of public health professionals: report of postal survey and discussion workshops*, West Midlands Cancer Intelligence Unit and NHS Executive West Midlands, Birmingham: Institute of Public and Environmental Health, University of Birmingham.

Somervaille, L. and Griffiths, R. (1998) 'Public health professionals, West Midlands Cancer Intelligence Unit and NHS Executive West Midlands follow up survey', Birmingham.

Somervaille, L., Knight, T. and Cornish, Y. (2007) 'A short history of the multidisciplinary public health forum', *Public Health*, vol 121, no 6, pp 409–13.

Taylor, S. and Coyle, E. (2001) 'For and against: public health does not need to be led by doctors. Education and debate', *British Medical Journal*, vol 322 (30 June), p 1595.

Todd Report (1968) *Royal Commission on Medical Education 1965–8*, Cm 3569, London: HMSO.

Wanless, D. (2002) *Securing our future health: taking a long-term view*, London: HM Treasury.

Wanless, D. (2004) *Securing good health for the whole population, final report*, 25 February, London: HM Treasury.

Warren, M. (1997) *The genesis of the Faculty of Community Medicine*, Canterbury: Centre for Health Services Studies, University of Kent at Canterbury.

Webster, C. (1996) *The health services since the war. Vol 2: government and health care – the British NHS 1958–79*, London: The Stationery Office.

Whittaker, M. and Barnes, G. (2005) 'There is an end to training', *Ph.com: The Newsletter of the Faculty of Public Health*, March, p 7.

WHO (World Health Organisation) (1981) *Global strategy for health for all by the year 2000*, Geneva.

WHO and United Nations International Children's Fund (UNICEF) (1978) *Statement at Alma Ata, primary health care*, Geneva.

WHO Europe (1986) *Ottawa Charter for health promotion*, First International Conference on Health Promotion, Geneva, October.

Winslow, C.E.A. (1923) *The evolution and significance of the modern public health*, New York, NY: Yale University Press.

Wright, J. (2007) 'Developing the public health workforce', in S. Griffiths and D. Hunter (eds) *New perspectives in public health*, Oxford: Radcliffe Publishing, pp 217–23.

Wright, J., Rao, M. and Walker, K. (2008) 'The UK public health skills and career framework – an opportunity to unite the multi-disciplinary, multi-agency workforce across EU states?', *Public Health*, vol 122, pp 541-4.

Wright, J., Dunkley, R. and Pittam, G. (2010) 'The role of the Directors of Public Health in England', unpublished study for the Association of Directors of Public Health, Public Health Resource Unit.

Wright, K. (2011) *An evaluation of the factors which led to the opening of the higher specialist training scheme for public health to those from a background other than medicine and its impact on the profile of public health specialists in England*, Masters in Public Health dissertation, King's College London.

Appendix 1: Timeline

This chronology has been adapted from the version presented within the Witness Seminar held in 2005 (Evans et al, 2006) on multidisciplinary public health and updated.

Year	Key events that had an impact on the development of a multidisciplinary public health workforce
1948	The National Health Service (NHS) began in the UK on 5 July. Local government retained the management of health centres, maternity and child welfare services, home nursing, health visiting, immunisation, other prevention work, and ambulance services under Medical Officers for Health. The new health service employed some public health doctors as medical administrators.
1968	The Royal Commission on Medical Education 1965–68 (Command 3569) recommended a period of general, followed by higher professional, training for all doctors following their internship year after graduation. It considered that there were sufficient elements in common for doctors between medical administration, social medicine and public health for these to be treated as a single specialty of community medicine. It recommended the setting up of a professional body to bring together academic and service interests in public health and assess professional training.
1970	The final proposal for a new 'Faculty of Community Medicine' (a faculty of the Royal College of Physicians) noted that, 'at a later date, and by agreement with the Royal Colleges, consideration would be given to the eligibility of non-medical colleagues practising, teaching or conducting research in the field of Community Medicine' (Warren, 1997, p 45) for membership of the Faculty.
1972	Publication of the Working Party on Medical Administrators (Hunter Report), which recommended that specialist postgraduate training for community medicine should include epidemiology, statistics, environmental health, social and behavioural sciences, social administration, and health services management.
	The Faculty of Community Medicine was created by the Royal Colleges of Physicians of Edinburgh and London and the Royal College of Physicians. Membership was restricted to registered medical practitioners.

1974	Implementation of new health and local government structures. The post of Medical Officer of Health was abolished. Public health doctors previously employed by local authorities were moved into the new district, area and regional health authority structures as specialists in community medicine and community physicians.
	Faculty of Community Medicine holds first examination for membership as the recognised specialist qualification.
1978	Declaration of Alma Ata, by the World Health Organization. Led to development of the Public Health Alliance and the Association for Public Health in UK.
1981	'Health for all by the year 2000' World Health Organization initiative.
1983	Publication of the NHS Management Inquiry Report (Griffiths Report). Led to ending of consensus-style management and the introduction of general management.
1986	Publication of the Inquiry Report following the outbreak of salmonella at Stanley Royd Hospital.
1988	Publication of *Public health in England: the report of the Committee of Inquiry into the Future Development of the Public Health Function* (Acheson, 1988), which identified public health as a multidisciplinary endeavour while retaining medical leadership. It also recommended that there should be a Director of Public Health (DPH) within each health district and region.
1989	The Faculty of Community Medicine changed its name to the Faculty of Public Health Medicine.
1990	NHS and Community Care Act, which led to the introduction of an internal market in the health service in England from April 1991.
	Establishment of multidisciplinary Masters in Public Health at Cardiff University.
1991	Creation of a category of 'Honorary Membership' at the Faculty of Public Health Medicine open to those in disciplines other than medicine.
1992	Masters in Public Health at the London School of Hygiene and Tropical Medicine opened to graduates from outside medicine.
1994	Survey of public health professionals identified over 1,500 people from backgrounds other than medicine working in public health in the UK.
1995	National seminar held in Birmingham to explore the career structures, training, accreditation and professional roles in multidisciplinary public health, followed by workshops across different English regions and UK nations to facilitate networking and explore education and development needs.

1996	Survey of members of the Faculty of Public Health Medicine, the majority of whom voted against opening examinations and full membership to disciplines other than medicine.
	Second national conference, 'Multidisciplinary Public Health – Moving Forward' organised, which led to the establishment of the Multidisciplinary Public Health Forum, with a National Core Group working through regional and national networks.
1997	Third national multidisciplinary public health conference in Birmingham, 'Multidisciplinary Public Health – What Next?'
	Joint 'Statement of Intent' from the Multidisciplinary Public Health Forum and Royal Institute of Public Health to work together on the development of a framework for the education, development and accreditation of multidisciplinary public health professionals.
1998	Multidisciplinary Public Health Forum 'Position Paper' on training, education, and accreditation of multidisciplinary public health.
	Chief Medical Officer's project to strengthen the public health function in England: a report of emerging findings (Calman, 1998) expressed commitment to developing multidisciplinary working.
	Successful vote of the membership of the Faculty of Public Health Medicine to open its Part I examination and diplomate membership to graduates from disciplines other than medicine.
	Faculty of Public Health Medicine joins with Multidisciplinary Public Health Forum and the Royal Institute of Public Health to form the Tripartite Group to work towards multidisciplinary accreditation.
1999	English White Paper *Saving lives: our healthier nation* (DH, 1999a) made a commitment to create a role of 'specialist in public health'. The Health Development Agency to replace the Health Education Authority.
	Fourth national multidisciplinary public health conference held in Bristol.
	First formal regional training schemes for non-medical specialists in public health established.
	First sitting of newly opened Part I Faculty examination.
	Feasibility study of the case for national standards for specialist practice in public health (Lessof et al, 1999) published.
2000	Secretary of State for Health's speech to the London School of Economics (Milburn, 2000) includes a call to 'take public health out of the ghetto' and end 'lazy thinking and occupational protectionism' in public health.

	Consultant-level specialist in public health posts open to disciplines other than medicine advertised by some Health Authorities.
2001	Publication of *Shifting the balance of power* (DH, 2001), which led to the creation of 303 Primary Care Trusts (PCTs) and 28 Strategic Health Authorities, each with a public health team with a board-level (DPH) appointment. 100 health authorities replaced.
	Announcement by Lord Hunt at the Faculty of Public Health Medicine Annual Lecture that 'this generation of directors of public health will be from a variety of backgrounds not only medical. This reform offers an opportunity to make multidisciplinary public health a reality' (Hunt, 2001).
	The first multidisciplinary public health trainee passed the Faculty Part I membership examination.
	At the Faculty's Annual General Meeting, the membership voted in favour of opening the membership to persons from a public health background other than medicine and making the Part II examination available to both medical and non-medical public health professionals.
	Publication of the final report of the Chief Medical Officer's project to strengthen the public health function categorised the public health workforce into three groups – specialists, practitioners and wider workforce.
	Formation of the UK Public Health Association from the Public Health Alliance, the Association for Public Health and the Public Health Trust.
	Publication of the *Public health skills audit* (Burke et al, 2001) included public health skills in organisational development and partnership-working.
2002	Faculty of Public Health Medicine Part II examination and full membership by examination opened to disciplines other than medicine.
	Appointment of first UK Directors of Public Health from backgrounds other than medicine in PCTs.
	Unfinished business (Donaldson, 2002) published, with proposals to reform the Senior House Officer medical grade, with consequences for public health specialist training, which were later realised as part of *Modernising medical careers* (DH, 2004a).
	Agreement on the 10 key areas of public health practice.
	The HM Treasury Wanless Report published, stating that the health service would become unaffordable if people did not take more responsibility for their own health.

2003	Establishment of UK Voluntary Register for Public Health Specialists with support from all four UK health departments. First registration through the retrospective portfolio assessment route.
	Faculty of Public Health Medicine's name changed to the Faculty of Public Health.
	The first multidisciplinary public health trainee passed the Faculty Part II membership examination.
	Start of Department of Health (DH)-supported top-up schemes in regions to support suitable senior public health professionals from backgrounds other than medicine to prepare portfolios to be assessed for registration.
	Funding from the DH of leadership schemes for public health in London and the West Midlands.
2004	The DH published, *Agenda for change: final agreement* (2004), which brought a new single pay scale for the NHS, and provided an opportunity to ensure equality in salaries for doctors and other public health specialists occupying Consultant in Public Health roles.
	Modernising medical careers: the next steps published by DH (2004a), beginning the programme to reform specialist (medical) training in public health.
	Skills for Health (2004) published the *National Occupational Standards for Public Health* based on the 10 key areas.
	The Nursing and Midwifery Council launched standards of proficiency for specialist community public health nurses as part of its new register.
	Choosing health (DH, 2004b) White Paper (government's response to the Wanless Report) signalled commitment to develop the whole of the public health workforce to help empower individuals to adopt healthier lifestyles. The new health trainer workforce launched.
2005	First trainee from a background other than medicine completes higher specialist training and registers on the UK Voluntary Register for Public Health Specialists.
2006	Reduction in the number of PCTs led to larger public health teams. Introduction of DsPH as joint appointments between health and local government.
	Agreement by national public health organisations on the four core areas of public health and five defined areas of practice.
	The UK Public Health Register invited applications for voluntary registration of defined specialists through retrospective portfolio assessment.

2007	Agenda for Change pay circular provides a national framework for pay and on-call remuneration for public health specialist trainees.
	All public health trainees became known as Specialty Registrars.
2008	National recruitment begins for multidisciplinary higher specialist training in public health.
	Publication by Skills for Health (2008) of the 'UK public health skills and career framework' based on four core areas and five defined areas of practice across nine career levels.
2010	The UK Public Health on-line Resource for Careers, Skills and Training in (PHORCaST) launched.
	Incoming Coalition government published its White Papers for NHS and public health reform.
	Report of review of regulation of public health specialists (DH, 2010c) recommends statutory regulation for generalist specialists. Case for defined specialists and practitioners not proven.
2011	Around a third of the current membership of the Faculty of Public Health are from backgrounds other than medicine, a proportion that will continue to rise.
	Since the UK Public Health Register opened in 2003, over 500 public health specialists registered, 107 of whom came through the 'standard' training scheme route.
	UK Public Health Register invites voluntary registration by retrospective portfolio assessment for practitioners in UK Public Health Register-approved pilot schemes.
2011	Single assessment centre used for recruitment to public health specialist training for the first time.
2012	*Outcomes framework for public health* (DH, 2012a) published.
	NHS Future Forum report advocates public health awareness across the NHS workforce. 'Making every contact count' programme launched in some health regions.
	NHS Health and Social Care Act passed, which changes health service structure and required upper-tier councils to set up Health and Wellbeing Boards to oversee strategic health and social care planning.
	Government sets target of recruiting 4,200 new health visitors in England by 2015.

2013	Implementation of new public health and NHS structures. Start of Public Health England as executive agency of the DH. Staff working on local health improvement programmes move from PCTs to upper-tier councils; DsPH joint appointments between the secretary of state and upper-tier councils. Two-year ring-fenced funding to upper-tier councils for the establishment of Health Education England and Local Education and Training Boards, with responsibility for the funding of education and training; some have formal public health representation. PHORCaST moves to HEE.
	Public health workforce strategy (DH et al, 2013) for England advocates feasibility study to look at setting up online skills passports for public health.
	DH consultation on statutory regulation arrangements for non-medical public health specialists.
	Scotland joined the national recruitment process for public health training.

Appendix 2: Glossary of terms

AAC	Advisory Appointments Committee	Statutorily required committee, with specified representation, including from the relevant Royal College, for the appointment of medical consultants in the UK National Health Service (NHS). For information on the consultant in public health appointments process visit, www.fph.org.uk
ADsPH	Association of Directors of Public Health	In current form since 1989. Representative body of Directors of Public Health across the UK. Aims to maximise effectiveness and impact of DsPH as public health leaders. Visit: www.adph.org.uk
AfC	Agenda for Change	Since 1 December 2004, the grading and pay system for all NHS staff apart from doctors, dentists and very senior managers.
ARCP	Annual Review of Competence Progression	Applies to specialist registrars on the public health training scheme.
AT	Area Team	From April 2013, 27 ATs accountable to NHS England; responsible for commissioning of independent contractor services, prison health, screening, under fives, tertiary care.
BMA	British Medical Association	Trade union and professional body for doctors.

CCG	Clinical Commissioning Group	Each of the 8,000 general practices in England is part of one of the 211 CCGs since 1 April 2013 responsible for commissioning of secondary and community health care. Overall, responsible for 60% of NHS budget.
CDC	Centers for Communicable Diseases and Prevention	The national public health institute of the United States. Based in Atlanta, Georgia.
CHRE	Council for Healthcare Regulatory Excellence	Established under the NHS Reforms and Healthcare Professions Act 2002 as an independent non-departmental public body to coordinate standards and good practice among the bodies responsible for regulating health care professionals in the UK.
CIEH	Chartered Institute of Environmental Health	Founded in 1883 to set standards, accredit courses and award qualifications for environmental health practitioners. Covers England, Northern Ireland and Wales.
CMO	Chief Medical Officer	The most senior advisor on health matters to the government. There is one CMO for each UK country. In England, the CMO is a civil servant and part of the Department of Health (DH). Not necessarily a public health doctor.
Coalition government	Current government in UK	In power since May 2010, formed of Conservatives and Liberal Democrats.

CPH	Consultant in public health	Senior public health post. Appointed by AAC to consultant post. Is on the specialist register for public health of the General Medical Council (GMC), General Dental Council (GDC) or UK Public Health Register (UKPHR).
Deanery	Deanery	Local structure responsible for management and delivery of postgraduate medical and dental education and continuing professional development (CPD). Part of new education structure of Health Education England.
DH	Department of Health	A department of the UK government with responsibility for health and social care and the NHS in England.
DHSSPS	Department of Health, Social Services and Public Safety for Northern Ireland	Part of Northern Ireland Executive, created by the Northern Ireland Act 1998. Responsible for health and social care.
DMS	Defence Medical Services	The DMS includes the Headquarters Surgeon General (HQSG), Joint Medical Command (JMC), Defence Dental Services (DDS) and the three single service (army, navy and air force) medical organisations. It is headed by the Surgeon General (SG). Medical, dental and related support services are provided to armed forces personnel by the Ministry of Defence (MOD), the NHS, charities and welfare organisations.

DNAC	Development Needs Assessment Centre 2003–06	Nationally coordinated support team to provide expertise to regional schemes for development of aspiring public health specialists preparing for portfolio registration with the UKPHR.
DPH	Director of Public Health	Strategic public health leader at the local level. In England since 1 April 2013, joint appointments between the secretary of state and upper-tier local authorities.
ECCH	European Centre for Connected Health, Belfast	Part of Public Health Agency in Northern Ireland. Uses technology to provide health care remotely.
EHO	Environmental health officer	Regulated with Chartered Institute of Environmental Health (CIEH) to deliver environmental health services in the public and private sectors.
Faculty advisor	Faculty advisor	Represents the Faculty of Public Health (FPH) as professional advisor on competency and qualifications of applicants and interviews for consultant in public health appointments.
FPH(M)	Faculty of Public Health (Medicine) and, between 1974 and 1989, Faculty of Community Medicine	The faculty of the Royal College of Physicians that acts as the standard-setting body for public health specialists from any background. Medicine was removed from the title in 2003.
GDC	General Dental Council	Regulatory body for dentists and dental health practitioners for the UK.
GMC	General Medical Council	Regulatory body for doctors for the UK.
GP	General Practitioner	Qualified physician, regulated with the GMC, offering primary care services to patients.

GPFH	GP Fundholding	Scheme established in the 1990s by the Conservative government to allow GPs to purchase elective secondary care for their patients. Disbanded by the Labour government in 1999.
Green Paper	Green Paper	Government report and consultation document on policy proposals.
HCPC	Health and Care Professions Council	UK regulator for health professionals apart from doctors and dentists.
HEA/HDA	Health Education Authority/Health Development Agency	HEA established in 1987 as a special health authority to encourage health education and health promotion. Replaced by the HDA in 2000 and then became part of the National Institute for Health and Care Excellence (NICE) in 2005.
Health and Social Care Act 2012	Health and Social Care Act 2012	Implemented in England on 1 April 2013 as part of the Coalition governments reforms to the health service, established CCGs, PHE and Health and Wellbeing Boards (HWBBs).
HealthWorkUK/ SfH	HealthWorkUK/Skills for Health	One of 25 Sector Skills Councils in the UK, responsible for health and the production of national occupational standards.
HEE	Health Education England	A special health authority created from April 2013 as part of the health service reforms to lead the education and training system in England for the health and public health workforce.

HPA	Health Protection Agency	Created as special health authority in April 2003 to provide an integrated approach to protecting UK public health. Became a non-departmental public body in April 2005 when it incorporated radiation protection. In England, it became part of Public Health England (PHE) on 1 April 2013.
HV	Health Visitor	Qualified public health nurse, registered with the Nursing and Midwifery Council (NMC) to provide advice and help within primary and community care to individuals, families and communities.
HWBB	Health and Wellbeing Boards	Established as part of the Coalition government's health reforms. Statutory boards led by upper-tier councils to provide oversight for local health and social care strategy, improve health, and reduce inequalities.
JCHMT	Joint Committee on Higher Medical Training	Hosted by Royal College of Physicians.
LA	Local authorities	Democratically run structures with devolved powers from central government to run local services, such as housing, education and planning, with a combination of central funding and locally raised council taxation of residents.
LETB	Local Education and Training Board	Twelve employer-led structures in England to lead planning and commissioning at the local level, authorised and hosted by HEE.

LGA	Local Government Association	Politically led, cross-party organisation to ensure that local government has a strong voice within central government.
MDPH	Multidisciplinary Public Health	Generic term used to mean those disciplines contributing to delivery of the public health function apart from medicine; also used to refer to the whole of the public health workforce, including doctors.
MECC	Making Every Contact Count	Initiative from NHS Future Forum report in 2012 calling for every contact with the public made by a health care professional to use the opportunity to help them improve their health.
MMC	Modernising Medical Careers	Policy issued for restructuring postgraduate medical training, education and organisation across the UK.
MoH	Medical Officer of Health	Local lead for health within local government from the mid-1880s until 1974, when such posts transferred to the NHS.
MoU	Memorandum of Understanding	Agreement across two or more parties where no legally binding arrangements exist.
MPET	Multi-professional Education and Training Budget	The bringing together into a single budget of health care training and development funds for doctors and dentists (Medical and Dental Levy – MADEL) and the non-medical workforce (Non-Medical Education and Training – NMET).
MSC	Modernising Scientific Careers	Strategy issued in February 2010 for the development of the UK health care scientific workforce, its education and training.

National Public Health Service for Wales (Public Health Wales)elath	National Public Health Service for Wales (Public Health Wales)	Public Health Wales was created as an NHS Trust in 2009 with statutory public health functions, including health protection and health care improvement. It replaced the National Public Health Service for Wales, which had existed since 2003.
NHS	National Health Service	System for centrally funded provision of health care for UK countries from 1948, free at the point of access.
NHS Education for Scotland	NHS Education for Scotland	Special health board responsible for developing and delivering education and training for those who work in NHS Scotland.
NHS England	NHS England	Non-departmental public body responsible for overseeing the commissioning of health care in England.
NHS Health Scotland	NHS Health Scotland	Special Health Board, national agency in NHS Scotland for improving health.
NHS Leadership Academy	NHS Leadership Academy	Funded from April 2013 to improve and develop leadership across the NHS in England.
NHS (Management) E	NHS (Management) Executive	Created in 1989 and disbanded in 2002. Provided overall management of the NHS and advice on health policy to ministers.
NHS Trust	NHS Trust (hospital and community services)	NHS (Foundation) Trusts are not-for-profit public benefit corporations providing services to patients.
NMC	Nursing and Midwifery Council	UK regulatory body for nurses and midwives
NMET	Non Medical Education and Training	National funding for the commissioning of education and training for health service staff apart from doctors.

Northern Ireland Assembly	Northern Ireland Assembly	Devolved legislature for Northern Ireland, making laws on all transferred matters.
Northern Ireland Executive	Northern Ireland Executive	Administrative branch of the Assembly, responsible for governance of Northern Ireland under the terms of the Good Friday Agreement.
OSPHE	Objective Structured Public Health Examination	'Show how' examination of FPH trainees to demonstrate competency in real-life situations.
PCT	Primary Care Trust	The statutory authority for commissioning of health care between 2002 and 2013.
PHE	Public Health England	Civil service agency for public health from April 2013, principally encompassing the HPA and centrally commissioned health intelligence functions.
PHSCF	Public Health Skills and Career Framework	Competency framework applying to the whole of the public health workforce (specialists, practitioners and the wider workforce), issued by Skills for Health and the Public Health Resource Unit.
PHWAG	Public Health Workforce Advisory Group	Advisory body on public health development and workforce issues to the DH, including representation from each UK country and national public health organisations.
PMETB	Postgraduate Medical Education Training Board	Merged with the GMC in April 2010.
Public Health Agency, Northern Ireland	Public Health Agency, Northern Ireland	Created in 2009 and responsible for public health improvement, health protection, health and social care commissioning advice, and research and development.

RCN	Royal College of Nursing	Professional organisation for all nurses in the UK.
RCP	Royal College of Physicians	One of the medical Royal Colleges; two in the UK – RCP London and Edinburgh; Joint Royal College of Physicians and Surgeons of Glasgow. Professional body responsible for standard-setting and overseeing the training of doctors practising in general and related medicine.
RDPH	Regional Director of Public Health	Strategic Director of Public Health. Civil service RDsPH replaced the previous NHS Regional Medical Officers in 1995.
RIPH/RSH/ RSPH	Royal Institute of Public Health/Royal Society of Health/Royal Society for Public Health	RSPH formed in 2008 from merger of the RIPH and the RSH as an independent charity to promote and protect human health and well-being: a membership organisation open to anyone in public health; provides policy advice, education and training services.
SHA	Strategic Health Authority	Statutory body created in 2002 to oversee local health services; 28 SHAs in 2002 reduced to 10 in 2006 and disbanded 2013.
SPH	Specialist in Public Health	Accredited at specialist level with the GMC, GDC or UKPHR. Eligible to apply for consultant in public health posts.
UKPHA	UK Public Health Association	Independent voluntary organisation formed in 1999 to unite the public health movement in the UK. Absorbed within the FPH in 2012.

UKPHR	UK Public Health Register	Created in 2003 as an independent voluntary register for the registration and regulation of public health specialists and, from 2011, for practitioners.
Wales Centre for Health	Wales Centre for Health	A Welsh Assembly-sponsored body created in 2005 to support development and training. Absorbed within Public Health Wales in 2009.
Welsh Assembly Government	Welsh Assembly Government	Devolved government for Wales.
White Paper	White Paper	Government policy.
WHO	World Health Organization	The public health arm of the United Nations; headquarters in Geneva.

Index

Note: The following abbreviations have been used – *f* = figure; *n* = note; *t* = table

Public health workforce strategy (England) (Department of Health) 108, 120, 124, 132, 135, 149, 151, 152–3, 170, 177
Public Sector Agreements (PSAs) 72
purchaser–provider split 155

Q

QCA *see* Qualifications and Curriculum Authority
Qualifications and Curriculum Authority (QCA) 67

R

Radiological Protection Board, National 61
Radiologists, Royal College of 44
RAE *see* Research Assessment Exercise
RCGP *see* Royal College of General Practitioners
RCN *see* Royal College of Nursing
RCP *see* Royal College of Physicians
RDsPH *see* Regional Directors of Public Health
'Record of in-Training Assessment' (RITA) 94, 98, 100
recruitment 95, 100–1, 102*f*, 103, 106
Reducing health inequalities: an action plan (Department of Health) 33*n*
REF *see* Research Assessment Exercise
Regional Directors of Public Health (RDsPH) 59, 60, 65, 76, 85, 92
  1990s public health movement 35, 39*n*, 40, 47, 48, 49
Regional Health Authorities 21, 34–5
Regional Service Provider Units 62
registration 57*n*, 67, 81, 83, 89, 122–4, 160
regulatory systems 89, 124, 148–9, 168–9
  defined specialists 83–4
  future of specialist regulation 84–6
  setting up 79–83
Report of an inquiry into the future development of the public health function in England (Acheson Report) 2, 7, 21*n*, 28–9, 33*n*, 34, 46
report of the Chief Medical Officer's project to strengthen the public health function in England, The (Donaldson) 63*n*, 124, 168
Research Assessment Exercise (RAE) (later Research Excellence Framework (REF)) 74*n*
RIPH *see* Royal Institute of Public Health and Hygiene
RITA *see* 'Record of in-Training Assessment'
Royal College of General Practitioners (RCGP) 143
Royal College of Nursing (RCN) 58–9, 66
Royal College of Pathologists 7*n*, 19, 20, 44
Royal College of Physicians (RCP) (London; Edinburgh) 19, 20, 44, 55, 107
Royal College of Radiologists 44
Royal College of Surgeons 107
Royal Commission on Medical Education (Todd Report) (1968) 17–18
Royal Institute of Public Health and Hygiene (RIPH) (later Royal Institute of Public Health) 41, 45*n*, 50, 74, 75*n*, 80, 81
Royal Society for the Promotion of Health (RSPH) 74, 75*n*
Royal Society for Public Health (RSPH) 147

S

salmonella 28
Sanitary Acts (1866–70) 1*n*
sanitation 16
SARS *see* Severe Acute Respiratory Syndrome
Saving lives: our healthier nation (Department of Health) 53–4, 56, 63*n*, 67, 89, 93, 112
Scally, Gabriel 85
scientists 37
Scotland 104, 55, 156*t*, 158–9, 177
Scottish Government Department for Health and Wellbeing 158
secondary care health service commissioners 32
Secretary of State for Health 134, 135, 139

Seebohm Report (*Report of the
  Committee on Local Authority and
  Allied Personal Social Services*)
  (1968) 17
Select Committee on Health 58, 59,
  62
Senior House Officers 100
senior public health professionals 22,
  53, 86
  academic public health 73–4
  categorisation of the workforce
    62–8
  Directors of Public Health 58–61
  formal partnerships and local
    authorities 72–3
  health protection agencies 61–2
  increasing public health capacity
    68–71
  National Health Service
    reorganisation 71–2
  non-medical public health specialists
    53–8
  progress at specialist level 74–7
  within local government 142–3,
    145*n*
Severe Acute Respiratory Syndrome
  (SARS) 2*n*, 10
Shape of Training review (2013) 109,
  167–8
*Shaping the future of public health:
  promoting health in the NHS*
  (Griffiths and Dark) 117
SHAs *see* Strategic Health Authorities
*Shifting the balance of power within the
  NHS: securing delivery* (Department
  of Health) 58, 80
skills audit 54
Skills for Health 65, 66*n*, 67, 112*n*,
  113, 117, 118, 122, 126, 151
Smith, Alwyn 25, 35
'snowballing' methodology 39–40
Social Exclusion Unit (Cabinet
  Office) 33*n*
Social Medicine, Society for (SSM)
  18–19
social work services: reorganisation 17
Society for Health 45*n*
Society of Health Education and
  Health Promotion Officers 27
Society of Medical Officers of Health
  18, 19

Society for Social Medicine (SSM)
  18, 19
Solutions for Public Health (SPH)
  120
Southgate Review 100
Special Health Boards (Scotland) 158
Specialist Development Committee
  (Faculty of Public Health
  Medicine) 56, 74
Specialist Register (General Medical
  Council) 79, 90
specialist trainees 95*n*, 97, 98–9, 101,
  102*f*, 103–4, 105*f*, 107–8, 109, 121
Specialist Training Coordinating
  Group (Faculty of Public Health
  Medicine) 98
specialists 1, 3*n*, 7, 11, 50, 62–8, 103,
  150, 163
  competency developments 67–8
  defined areas of practice 113–16
  defined specialists 83–4, 104, 115*n*,
    121, 122, 123, 152, 157, 168
  development of 17–20, 21*n*, 22–4
  hospitals 16
  public health role in National
    Health Service (NHS) 54
Specialists in Community Medicine
  (SCM) 21, 23*n*, 26
SPH *see* Solutions for Public Health
SSM *see* Society for Social Medicine
Stanley Royd Hospital 28
*Statement on managed public health
  networks* (Public Health and
  Primary Care Group (Faculty of
  Public Health Medicine)/Health
  Development Agency (HDA) 64
Strategic Health Authorities (SHAs)
  58, 59, 61, 71, 116, 128, 132
Surgeon General (US) 9
surgeons 16
Surgeons, Royal College of 107

T

teaching hospitals 16*n*
Teaching Public Health Networks,
  Association of (ATPHN) 126
Teaching Public Health Networks
  (TPHNs) 125–6, 151
'technical experts' 125
Todd Report (Royal Commission on
  Medical Education) (1968) 17–18